RURAL HEALTHCARE AND THE PANDEMIC

RURAL HEALTHCARE AND THE PANDEMIC

CHALLENGES, SOLUTIONS, AND FUTURE NEEDS

Dayle Sharp, Judith Paré, and Polly Petersen

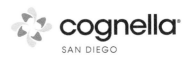

Bassim Hamadeh, CEO and Publisher
Amanda Martin, Executive Publisher
Amy Smith, Senior Project Editor
Maddie Lopez, Editorial Associate
Casey Hands, Production Editor
Jessica Delia, Graphic Design Associate
Kylie Bartolome, Licensing Specialist
Natalie Piccotti, Director of Marketing
Kassie Graves, Senior Vice President, Editorial

Cover image: Cover image generated using Adobe Firefly.
Interior image generated using Adobe Firefly.

Printed in the United States of America.

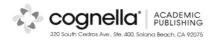
cognella® | ACADEMIC PUBLISHING
320 South Cedros Ave., Ste. 400, Solana Beach, CA 92075

BRIEF CONTENTS

DETAILED CONTENTS

PREFACE

Utilizing Rural Nursing Theory as a Foundation for Rural Nursing Practice

To better understand rural nursing, one must understand rural residents' values. According to Long and Weinert (2022), rural dwellers value work and health beliefs differently from suburban or urban dwellers. For these citizens, maintaining a work ethic, or fulfilling one's work duties, is a core value. Rural dwellers measure a state of health in relation to work, role, and work functions, and health needs are almost always secondary to work needs. These residents also highly value self-reliance and independence. The desire to be independent and care for one's needs independently influences the health-seeking behaviors of rural residents. Each of these values has implications for all healthcare providers and nurses practicing in rural areas and can provide role modeling for nurses new to rural and remote settings.

Long and Weinert (2022) emphasize that the stresses that affect nurses and their nursing practice are exceptionally significant. Rural nurses frequently describe themselves as being isolated from their urban and suburban colleagues. They frequently encounter patient care situations in which there is little or no support from colleagues to guide them in defining their scope of practice and its limitations. In the rural United States, most bedside nurses possess an Associate of Science in Nursing. This provides the skills needed by a nurse generalist but does not provide a strong foundation in change theory and leadership (Long & Weinert, 2022). There also remains a gap in the availability of an extensive orientation program in most rural areas that would instill competency in nurses for accessing current and diverse sources of best-practice information.

Long and Weinert (2022) state that nursing must address two specific aspects of rural culture: a nonjudgmental approach for those who delay treatments and a strong emphasis on sharing knowledge of preventive health practices that will allow individuals to remain independent and productive members of their communities. Therefore, the nurse's primary role involves providing education, support, and relief for family members, friends, and neighbors, who are often the main support for residents who are ill or have a disability. The nurse's success in achieving acceptance and trust in their role will require extended time; involvement in community activities, such as local civic or church activities; and the community's acknowledgment that the nurse is a welcome member. This is important as we look at times of not only overwhelming health crisis but also crises in rural communities' day-to-day life.

Authors' Note

All case studies presented in this text are the result of many interviews conducted with various professional healthcare providers and leaders as well as community leaders across the United States who provided the authors with powerful and invaluable reflection, thoughts, and ideas of their experiences throughout the COVID-19 period from 2020 to 2023. These people shared one focus: to keep patients, family, and friends safe, no matter what challenges they encountered.

Reference

Long, K. A., & Weinert, C. (2022). Rural nursing theory: Developing the theory base. In C. A. Winters (Ed.), *Rural nursing: Concepts, theory, and practice* (6th ed., pp. 13–23). Springer Publishing.

REVIEWERS

Ann M. Bowling, PhD, APRN, CPNP-PC, CNE, CHSE
Wright State University
Dayton, Ohio

Amanda L. Fischer, PhD, RN
Waynesburg University
Waynesburg, Pennsylvania

Mary Ann Glendon, PhD, RN
Southern Connecticut State University
New Haven, Connecticut

Angeline Bushy, PhD, RN, LTC, U.S. Army (Ret.)
University of Central Florida, College of Nursing
Orlando, Florida

Policy

The Impact and the Changes

Numerous state and federal policies dictate how health care is delivered in the United States. However, in most states, these policies and regulations were set aside to facilitate the care of the significant number of sick people with COVID-19. The areas in which these changes occurred included scope of practice, licensure of healthcare professionals, the Emergency Medical Treatment and Labor Act, certificates of need, and changes in areas of provision of direct patient care, clinical trial protocols, and other research opportunities that contribute to epidemiology and cure of a disease (Centers for Medicare & Medicaid Services, 2023). Capabilities of facilities collaborating for better patient outcomes and effective use of the healthcare workforce also resulted from changes in regulations. However, the division between citizens who disagreed on Centers for Disease Control and Prevention recommendations regarding mask mandates and immunizations contributed to increased infection rates that have never been seen before in the United States or the world.

Reference

Centers for Medicare & Medicaid Services. (n.d.). *Emergency Medical Treatment & Labor Act (EMTALA)*. https://www.cms.gov/Regulations-and-Guidance/ Legislation/EMTALA

CHAPTER 1

Rural Health Leadership Response to the 2020 Pandemic

Rural hospitals across the United States face precarious times. When these facilities were confronted with a situation in which their resources were stretched beyond their limits, the only solution appeared to be to shutter their doors. State and federal policies and regulations, financial challenges, and human resources were areas that many stand-alone critical access hospitals (CAHs) (Centers for Medicare & Medicaid Services [CMS], 2023) found extremely challenging. CAHs are found in rural areas and qualify for this designation by following federal guidelines that include having a location that is either more than 35 miles from the nearest hospital or more than 15 miles in areas of mountainous terrain or only secondary roads; having no more than 25 inpatient beds; holding acute inpatients for no longer than 96 hours, at which time patients must be discharged or transferred to a larger tertiary center; and providing 24-hour emergency care services seven days per week (CMS, 2023). Leadership knowledge, creativity, and flexibility were also challenged during the time of the pandemic and continue to require commitment to the mission of rural health care.

Leadership responses in acute care situations varied across the country. When nurses were asked about support during the COVID-19 surges, some said they felt they had complete support of their managers and hospital administration. Other nurses found themselves in circumstances that challenged their professional and ethical core as a result of perceived lack of support from their leaders. This support manifested itself in lack of resources such as personal protective equipment (PPE) (Occupational Safety & Health Administration, n.d.) allocated to personnel who provided direct, hands-on patient care; apparent disproportionate wages and benefits such as housing and wages provided to traveling nurses; and inconsistent patient assignments. Some facilities utilized federal funding to pay salary dollars to employees rather than initiate a reduction in force or layoffs. As a result of entire unit shutdowns, such as surgical services, especially for elective, nonemergency procedures, some staff were given no choice but to become oriented to providing care in intensive care or emergency departments. Some agencies utilized this option to coerce staff to either retrain for a different unit from which they currently worked in or seek alternative employment or retirement. Many hospitals in urban areas revamped their delivery of care to focus on the large percentage of COVID-19 patients. Entire units were created in atypical settings, and many bedside caregivers were retrained to care for severely sick patients, such as those on ventilators with extensive pharmacologicals and needing dialysis and multiple interventions, all without support staff.

In rural settings, this was not an option. CAHs typically transfer patients that are critically ill to larger tertiary centers. Therefore, staff have limited experiences taking care of acutely ill patients with these circumstances. Caring for the complex COVID-19 patients led to significant increases in anxiety for many rural healthcare providers. The World Health Organization (WHO) reported that at least 25% of healthcare workers reported anxiety, depression, and burnout symptoms (WHO, 2022). A mixed-methods study by the National Council of State Boards of Nursing (NCSBN) in 2023 confirmed that approximately 100,000 registered nurses (RNs) and 34,000 licensed practical and vocational nurses had left their positions since 2020 due to the COVID-19 pandemic (Smiley et al., 2023). When one-quarter of all nurses suffer from these symptoms and more than 134,000 nursing caregivers leave the healthcare workforce, leadership must reassess their commitment to those who provide acute bedside care. Leaders must earn the respect of their staff through commitment and decision-making that benefits the greater good, by putting at the forefront that which is best for many, and by setting aside their own needs. This type of leadership will influence the trust that healthcare providers have for administration when everyday life becomes chaotic, as it did throughout the COVID-19 pandemic.

Government Regulation Versus Healthcare Realities

Health care is an industry that is highly regulated by the government. Many rules and regulations affect multiple aspects within health care, such as the licensure of healthcare professionals, scope of practice of licensed providers, the number of patient beds and designations, staff-to-patient ratios, length of stay for patients in a rural CAH, and transfer criteria between facilities. Lack of skilled nursing facilities was an obstacle to the discharge of patients from the tertiary facility who were stable yet unable to be discharged home (Tamkin, 2022). Policies developed with healthcare providers' input have the potential to reduce stress, support recovery, and decrease workforce shortages (Limoges et al., 2022). However, during the COVID-19 crisis, many of these rules and regulations were put aside to facilitate care. "The resilience of health systems is relevant when facing any crisis, whether it be a sudden event like a tsunami, an evolving challenge such as antimicrobial resistance, or an enduring issue like medicines shortages, even without a sudden health crisis like the COVID-19 pandemic" (Hill et al., 2020, p. 294).

COVID-19 led to many healthcare facilities facing staffing shortages. Many providers became ill themselves, and the depth of backup was just not a reality. COVID-19 also led to many new staffing patterns and innovations (Tamkin, 2022). Licensure of healthcare workers was another area that changed dramatically. Typically, RNs, doctors, and respiratory therapists are licensed to practice through a state agency or board. However, as a result of either governor proclamations or those by state licensing agencies, flexibility in practice license by state was relaxed. Nurses who were licensed could practice legally in other states, even if the state was not a participant in the Nurse Licensure Compact, administered by the NCSBN. This was particularly important for those facilities that utilized a large number of travel nurses. Faced with a nursing shortage and education programs with limited access to clinical opportunities, 14 states allowed for nursing students to graduate early, take the

National Council Licensure Examination, and enter the workforce (Smith & Farra, 2022). Nurses who needed to renew a license to practice were given an extension, with some renewals delayed for a year.

Federal Policies in Direct Conflict With State Policies

Many federal policies and regulations were changed to try to reduce the rapid spread of COVID-19. Early in the pandemic, the Centers for Disease Control and Prevention (CDC) suggested mask mandates for anyone in a public place as well as canceling large gatherings such as sports activities and theater performances and social distancing to slow this spread. However, as COVID-19 became more politicized, many state officials across the United States suggested that there was no need for such dramatic actions. When a vaccination became available, many federal healthcare agencies required vaccinations for their employees.

CASE STUDY 1.1

Many state and federally funded hospitals were required to mandate COVID-19 vaccinations, which had an impact on nursing staffing. In one hospital, many of the nurses were of Eastern European descent, and due to their religious beliefs, they applied for religious exemptions. However, the state and hospital mandated that they be vaccinated. There was no allowance, either medical or religious, through which nurses were exempt from getting the vaccination. As a result, many staff resigned from the facility.

Many issues surrounding vaccination continue to exist. The state in which this hospital is located no longer enforces the rules requiring COVID-19 vaccination. Now the hospital is hiring nurses and providers who have not received this type of vaccination.

Consider that at the beginning of the pandemic and before the mandate, all nurses needed to be vaccinated, as many were caring for patients with COVID-19. The vaccination requirements came out after the fact that nurses had been caring for COVID-19 patients for a year without having been vaccinated. However, that reality suddenly changed once a vaccine had become available. The nurses were willing to stay but they didn't want to get the immunization for a variety of reasons; they understood the risk.

Vaccination

The controversy with mandatory vaccination brought to the forefront the individual's choice to vaccinate versus CDC recommendations and state and federal mandates for many in the healthcare field. For many years, healthcare facilities nationwide have required that healthcare workers be vaccinated for certain diseases to reduce outbreaks of vaccine-preventable illnesses. In some instances, facilities established these requirements due to mandates in state statutes and regulations. While they were often required to reduce the facilities' liability, they were usually the result of patient safety. But initial information about the development of vaccines for COVID-19, its effectiveness, and the political climate created doubt for many, including those in health care.

As of February 2022, there were 25 states that required vaccination for healthcare employees. Of those states, seven required boosters or current vaccination status; 21 states had requirements for healthcare workers to be vaccinated or regular testing for unvaccinated employees; and six states took the "vaccinate-or-terminate" approach with the exception of individuals who had valid religion or medical exemptions. Alternatively, 13 states passed laws banning employers from mandating vaccinations for employees (see Table 1.1).

TABLE 1.1 Vaccination Requirements for Healthcare Workers by State

Vaccination Requirements	State
Mandated boosters or up-to-date vaccine status	California, Connecticut, Massachusetts, New Jersey, New Mexico, New York
Mandated vaccination or termination	Colorado, Maine, New York, Oregon, Rhode Island, Washington
Mandated vaccination or testing	California*; Washington, D.C.; Delaware; Kentucky; Maryland*; Michigan; Nevada; New Jersey*; New Mexico*; North Carolina; Pennsylvania; Vermont; Wisconsin
Mandated vaccination or testing and masking	Connecticut,* Illinois, Maryland
Banned vaccination mandates for employees	Arizona, Arkansas, Florida, Georgia, Idaho, Indiana, Kansas, Montana, New Hampshire, North Dakota, Tennessee, Texas, Utah

*Healthcare workers with a valid religion or medical exemption.

Source: Pekruhn and Abbasi (2022).

Additional requirements at the federal level mandated that all healthcare employees working in federally funded facilities such as a veterans' hospital or clinic be vaccinated. This was sometimes in complete opposition to the vaccination rules within the state where the facilities were located. The mandates affected all CMS staff who worked in facilities and received Medicare and Medicaid payments (see Table 1.2).

TABLE 1.2 Types of CMS Facilities

Ambulatory surgery service	End-stage renal facilities
Ambulatory clinicals	Home infusion therapy services
Rehabilitation agencies	Hospices
Physical therapy and speech-language services	Hospitals
Community mental health centers	Intermediate care facilities
Outpatient rehabilitation centers	Long-term care facilities
Critical access hospitals	Psychiatric treatment facilities
Home health agencies	Rural health clinics/federally qualified health centers

Source: Centers for Medicare & Medicaid Services (2023).

Facilities met this mandate through two phases: Phase 1 required the facilities to have all policies and procedures in place to ensure all staff were fully vaccinated. Staff included in this phase had to receive the first dose of the primary series or a single dose of a COVID-19 vaccine prior to providing care, treatment, or other services in the facility. Phase 2 requirements mandated that all staff be fully vaccinated except for those who were granted an exception for religious reasons or due to having a history of vaccination allergy. This requirement was enforced by CMS' on-site surveys, which included the following criteria:

1. Plan for vaccinating all eligible staff to meet all thresholds
2. Plan to provide accommodations to those who were exempt
3. Plan for tracking and documenting staff vaccinations

A healthcare facility was out of compliance and subject to citations if all the above criteria were not met, although it was given the option to come into compliance. However, facilities that did not do so risked losing Medicare and Medicaid payments (CMS, 2023).

Conclusion

A multipronged, consistent approach involving all levels of health care will be required to address the unintended consequences of the COVID-19 pandemic effectively and proactively. National and international healthcare leaders must come together to commit to standards that illuminate issues of vaccine hesitancy, treatments for COVID-19, and physical and behavioral long-term support for residents and healthcare workers who continue to live with continued COVID-19 outbreaks and complications of the virus. Financial and technological support to advance the recruitment and retention of front-line healthcare workers will be essential to the survival of rural and remote healthcare settings. Additionally, long-term behavioral health support networks must be created and funded through state and national resources to support the needs of nurses who are struggling with the traumas they experienced during the first two years of the global pandemic.

Questions for Discussion Related to Case Study 1.1

1. Why were hospitals laying off or firing nurses who did not want to be vaccinated? Please consider all aspects of mandating vaccinations.
2. Why were the nurses told that they were not good enough because they declined to receive the vaccination? In what ways could nurses have been supported in their decision to decline getting the vaccination?

References

Centers for Medicare & Medicaid Services. (2023). Information for critical access hospital. *Medical Learning Network Booklet.* https://www.cms.gov/files/document/mln006400-information-critical-access-hospitals.pdf

Centers for Medicare and Medicaid Services. (2023). *COVID-19 vaccination requirements for health care providers and suppliers.* https://www.cms.gov/files/document/covid-19-health-care-staff-vaccination-requirements-infographic.pdf

Hill, R., Butnoris, M., Dowling, H., Macolina, K., Patel, B., Simpson, T., & Trevillian, S. (2020). Reflection on our leadership during COVID-19: Challenging our resilience. *Journal of Pharmacy Practice and Research, 50*, 291–296.

Limoges, J., McLean, J., Anzola, D., & Kolla, N. J. (2022). Effects of the COVID-19 pandemic on healthcare providers: Policy implications for pandemic recovery. *Healthcare Policy, 17*(3), 49–64.

Occupational Safety & Health Administration. (n.d.). *Personal protective equipment.* https://www.osha.gov/personal-protective-equipment

Pekruhn, D., & Abbasi, E. (2022). Vaccine mandates by state: Who is, who isn't, and how? Leading Age. https://leadingage.org/vaccine-mandates-by-state-who-is-who-isnt-and-how/

Smith, S. J., & Farra, S. L. (2022). The impact of COVID-19 on the regulation of nursing practice and education. *Teaching and Learning in Nursing, 17*, 302–305.

Smiley, R. A., Allgeyer, R. L., Shobo, Y., Lyons, K. C., Letourneau, R., Zhong, E., Kaminski-Orturk, N., & Alexander, M. (2023). The 2022 National Nursing Workforce Survey. *Journal of Nursing Regulation, 14*(1), S1–S90.

Tamkin, G. (2022). *Don't Waste the COVID Crisis: As the U.S. heads back to normal, we should never return to the old way health systems were run.* MedPage Today, Perspectives section https://www.medpagetoday.com/search?q=Don%27t+Waste+the+COVID&submit-button=/perspectives

World Health Organization. (2022). *World failing in 'our duty of care' to protect mental health and well-being of health and care workers, finds report on impact of COVID-19.* https://www.who.int/news/item/05-10-2022-world-failing-in--our-duty-of-care--to-protect-mental-health-and-wellbeing-of-health-and-care-workers--finds-report-on-impact-of-covid-19#:~:text=The%20report%20found%20that%2023.

CHAPTER 2

The Value of Leadership During a Pandemic

Many healthcare systems were not prepared for the resources needed to withstand the onslaught of patients infected with COVID-19. They did not have the workforce, supplies, or fiduciary depth. Additionally, continuous misinformation was provided from several sources every day, meaning that leaders had to deal with many issues that were unfamiliar to them. Thus, leadership was ill equipped and became ineffective. As nurses served on the front lines of healthcare surges, it became apparent that change needed to happen quickly and effectively. When those changes did not happen, nursing professionals who were overwhelmed by their circumstances of providing direct patient care were disgruntled and unhappy about their working conditions. It is estimated that two-thirds of all nurses will leave nursing within the next three years (Firth, 2022), adding to an already unprecedented nursing shortage. Leadership at all levels of an organization requires honesty, trust building, accountability, and a sense of community (Dowling & Kenney, 2020). According to one Swedish study, two main categories identified by employees related to the COVID-19 pandemic included concerns about exposure, potential infection, and reinfecting others, including family members, coworkers, and patients (Rücker et al., 2021). The impact of leadership played a significant role as the United States worked through and continued to adapt to living with COVID-19.

Nursing executives and leaders were challenged with innovative ways to address mistrust of healthcare systems, disgruntled staff, and unprecedented staffing shortages. More than one-half of respondents to an International Council of Nurses survey noted that nurses were asked to perform duties that were not within their scope of practice (Langan et al., 2022). Many nurses were asked to become intensive care unit nurses and manage patients on ventilators, multiple medication infusions, and end-of-life circumstances. According to findings from a 2022 qualitative study involving interviews of nurse executives at hospitals in the northeastern United States, the following six themes were identified that related to strategies and approaches to best support responses to the COVID-19 pandemic:

1. Redeploying, retraining, and regrouping clinical staff
2. Creating care team support roles

3. Meeting staffing needs
4. Recognizing nurse practitioners' skills in value-added, expanded functions
5. Emphasizing communication
6. Prioritizing mental health (Langan et al., 2022)

CASE STUDY 2.1

Hospital administration leadership styles vary. When administrators work together for the hospital and community, there are positive outcomes. At one critical access hospital (CAH), the chief nursing officer (CNO) and chief executive officer (CEO) worked together to make decisions during the pandemic. This allowed the CNO to discuss and support nursing issues and the CEO to speak to hospital finances. As a CNO, Jane was responsible for the nursing staff and ensuring there was adequate nursing coverage for the entire hospital for patient safety. She needed to review the daily census and patient diagnoses to guarantee she had nurses skilled in the care needed. In addition, she also needed to confirm she had the necessary support staff, such as certified nursing assistants and axillary staff. The CEO, Jeff, needed to ensure the hospital remained financially secure during the pandemic and to guarantee that all staff and patients had the resources they needed. When the two executives worked together, they were able to see both sides and make the best decision for all parties.

Leadership Styles

Because the arrival of COVID-19 was so quick and its transmission was so contagious, the virus' spread was rapid. This perfect storm resulted in the need for adaptation at all levels. Disaster plans that were previously planned and practiced no longer applied. Organizational charts were often inappropriate as many managers and leaders chose to lead externally from facilities, which resulted in a void that needed to be filled by those on the front lines of caring for the influx of patients. This resulted in many forms of leadership traits that were dictated by the circumstances. Healthcare professionals with no prior experience were empowered to step up and fill a leadership void, and that direction took on many forms. The support of nurse leaders was vital, with a direct correlation of staff commitment to ongoing patient care in the face of overwhelming working conditions. Effective nursing leadership can influence staff nurse recruitment, retention, job satisfaction, and commitment to the quality of patient care (Asiri et al., 2016). Leadership varied, based on previous leadership styles, prior experience, or behaviors and characteristics possessed by many immigrant leaders. The defined leadership approaches included *transformational, transactional, servant, relational*, and *hierarchical*.

Transformational Leadership

Transformational leadership is a model that nursing utilizes frequently to motivate staff to accept the greater good for the patient as well as the nursing unit. The leader does this by appealing to the followers' moral values and high ideals. The four components of transformational leadership are idealized influence, inspirational motivation, intellectual stimulation, and individualized consideration (Doody & Doody, 2012). Despite the overwhelming workload that healthcare professionals, particularly nurses, assumed during the pandemic, many respected the responsibility they had to the profession, their patients, and their community, all supported by the transformational leadership model.

Transactional Leadership

Leaders who focus on the transactional leadership model often utilize incentives and rewards for the types of behavior or actions appropriate for high-quality patient care. Transactional leaders take corrective action when monitoring their followers to promote effective task completion with tangible benefits and rewards for optimal performance (Harrington, 2021). Although many leaders believed they supported their staff's work during the pandemic with offerings of food and other small gifts, nurses shared that they eventually became tired of these types of incentives. Transactional leaders are effective in short-term crisis management because of their talents in shifting resources and personnel to address critical shortages. However, this style has been identified as one that minimizes the human factors related to prolonged stress and grief. The months and years since the beginning of the COVID-19 pandemic have necessitated a reexamination of transactional leadership in order to better address the workforce's fatigue and fragility. Many nurses felt that in utilizing this model, their leader overlooked both the physical and the mental wellness of staff. This consistent message also supports the fact that the nurses reported their own personal neglect of primary healthcare needs, including newly diagnosed illness and chronic health issues.

Servant Leadership

Leadership is difficult, complex, and multifaceted. The consequences of ineffective leadership can result in a deep impact on retention, a fact reported by a 2015 Gallup study indicating that 7,200 people had left their jobs due to their managers. Leadership is responsible for leading an organization to a desired future state while simultaneously keeping in sight the organization's mission and goals. Leadership requires a deep understanding of each individual's role in the organization's mission and vision. A leader must have an understanding of the roles of all employees as well as their common goal. Gandolfi and Stone (2016) defined *leadership* as "an intentional means by which a leader influences a group of people in an organization to a widely understood future state that is different from the present one." There are two guiding principles of leadership: "Everyone has some capacity to form leadership relationships, and leaders are made and not born" (Gandolfi & Stone, 2018, p. 264).

Servant executive leadership is a type of executive leadership that focuses on serving versus being served. The servant leader strives to work with each employee to reach their highest potential by creating a comfortable environment (The Black Sheep, 2022). Servant leadership incorporates 10 important characteristics: listening, empathy, healing, awareness, persuasion, conceptualization, foresight, stewardship, commitment to growth of people, and community building (Gandolfi & Stone, 2018, p. 265). Servant leadership focuses first on the ability for individuals to succeed and then the success of the organization's mission. Servant leaders achieve their goals by being proactive, ambitious, and driven and focusing on putting the follower first.

Complex Relational Leadership

Nurses are the largest population within the healthcare system, a fact that positions them to take the lead in leadership. Complex relational leadership (CRL) is a leadership model and conceptual framework that moves the paradigm of leadership from the leader-subordinate focus toward a transformational leadership, with relationships occurring between people and organizations. CRL focuses on nurses leading not from the top down but as collaborators working with other nurses and team members to enhance the organization's adaptability. CRL enables a professional governance framework in which leaders and clinical nurses collaborate to solve practice issues. CRL is described in three focus areas: professional governance, equitable and inclusive relationships, and clinical practice (Feistritzer et al., 2022, p. 145).

Executive Leadership

During and after the height of the pandemic surges, the U.S. healthcare system was faced with uncertainty and volatility, which required effective leaders. Executive leaders had the skills to guide the healthcare system through this difficult time. Executive leadership takes a controlled and systematic approach (The Black Sheep, 2022). This type of leader has clear goals for their organization and is skillful at adapting to situations by identifying the best course of action for the organization's healthcare workers. "The number one way to address the need for health care surge is to ensure that community-based interventions are maximally applied. This needs to be more effectively messaged to the community at large" (National Academies of Sciences, Engineering, and Medicine, 2020, p. 4). This is an excellent time to include community leaders by asking for their support to keep everyone in their rural community healthy and safe and making them aware of staffing levels, patient loads, and acuity.

Conclusion

In the presence of COVID-19, it is apparent that healthcare leaders must develop and implement strategies that address a different type of health care due to the endemic nature of the virus and other potentially life-threatening diseases that can become catastrophic. Simultaneously, there must also be strategies to care for many who have developed long-term complications from COVID-19. "Nurses appreciate the past, but there is no going back; innovation, listening to nurses' needs, and providing nurse support are the goals for a new normal" (Langan et al., 2022, p. E14).

Questions for Discussion Related to Case Study 2.1

1. Should rural CNOs and CEOs have roles in community engagement as a means of strengthening recruitment and retention of hospital staff? What roles should they assume, and what leadership style would be conducive to community engagement? Please explain your response and provide at least two examples.
2. Should rural CEOs actively recruit community members for positions on their hospital boards to better understand the physical, emotional, and financial impact of the COVID-19 pandemic on residents? If so, what methods could a rural CEO use to recruit hospital board members? For example, who might be the local stakeholders with whom rural CEOs should engage?

References

Asiri, S. A., Rohrer, W. W., Al-Surimi, K., Da'ar, O. O., & Ahmed, A. (2016). The association of leadership styles and empowerment with nurses' organizational commitment in an acute health care setting: a cross-sectional study. *BMC Nursing, 15*(38), 1–10.

Doody, O., & Doody, C. M. (2012). Transformational leadership in nursing practice. *British Journal of Nursing, 21*(20), 1212–1218.

Dowling, M. J., & Kenney, C. (2020). *Leading through a pandemic.* Skyhorse Publishing.

Feistritzer, N. R., Jackson, G., Scott, C., & Willis, P. (2022). Complex relational leadership: Meeting the challenge of post pandemic professional governance. *Nursing Administration Quarterly, 46*(2), 144–153. https://doi.org/10.1097/NAQ.0000000000000519

Firth, S. (2022). *Can virtual nursing save the workforce?* MedPage Today. https://www.med-pagetoday.com/nursing/nursing/101924?xid=nl_mpt_Nursing.update_2022-11-24 & eun=g1918045d0r&utm_source

Gandolfi, F., & Stone, S. (2016). Clarifying leadership: High-impact leaders in a time of leadership crisis. *Review of International Comparative Management, 17*(3), 212–224.

Gandolfi, F., & Stone, S. (2108). Leadership, leadership styles, and servant leadership. *Journal of Management Research, 18*(4), 261–269.

Harrington, A. (2021). Understanding effective nurse leadership styles during the COVID-19 pandemic. *Nursing Standard, 36*(5), 45–50.

Langan, J. C., Griffin, A. R., Shipman, S., & Dobalian, A. (2022). Nurse executive experiences with COVID-19: Now we know—we are not going back. *Nursing Administration Quarterly, 46*(2), E8–E15.

National Academies of Sciences, Engineering, and Medicine. (2020). *Rapid expert consultation on staffing considerations for crisis standards of care for the COVID-19 pandemic.* National Academies Press. https://doi.org/10.17226/25890

Rücker, F., Hårdstedt, M., Rücker, S. C. M., et al. (2021). From chaos to control—Experiences of healthcare workers during the early phase of the COVID-19 pandemic: A focus group study. *BMC Health Services Research, 21*, 1219. https://doi.org/10.1186/s12913-021-07248-9

The Black Sheep. (2022, November 30). *What is executive leadership? Types of executive leaders.* https://www.theblacksheep.community/executive-leadership/

Access to Care

Access to healthcare services is critical to good health. However, rural residents face various access barriers. Some of these include a lack of finances to support healthcare services, a lack of access to healthcare related to transportation, a lack of confidence in the healthcare they are provided, and a lack of trust in healthcare services that might result in a compromise of their privacy (Rural Health Information Hub, 2021). In addition to these obstacles, rural residents must face the dilemma of whether to go to work or attend a medical appointment as many of them have no paid time off. Many also have physical limitations or acute conditions; rural Americans are older, sicker, and poorer than their urban counterparts (Rural Health Information Hub, 2021). Other challenges include the lack of providers, stability of rural hospitals and clinics, or appropriate staffing for critical access hospitals.

Reference

Rural Health Information Hub. (2022). *Healthcare access in rural communities*. https://www.ruralhealthinfo.org/topics/healthcare-access

CHAPTER 3

The Challenges and Opportunities of Rural Health Care

Access to healthcare services is critical to optimal health (Rural Health Information Hub [RHIhub], 2021). Overall, rural populations are older and sicker than their urban counterparts and face an increasing gap in life expectancy. Public health emergencies such as the coronavirus (COVID-19) pandemic have exacerbated these disparities. Janke et al. (2021) found that hospital resources, including intensive care beds, nurses, and medical/surgical beds, were all statistically significantly associated with higher COVID-19 death rates. Many rural facilities struggle with each of these resources, especially if they are a standalone facility, or one unaffiliated with a larger system hospital or clinic. Rural communities also face a variety of access barriers, including chronic workforce shortages (Council on Graduate Medical Education, 2020), distance and transportation problems, limited health insurance coverage and broadband access, social stigma, and privacy issues (RHIhub, 2021).

Workforce Shortages

Workforce shortages in rural areas have existed for decades, a problem that increased during the pandemic. A large portion of rural America has been declared medically underserved (U.S. Department of Health and Human Services, n.d.) by the U.S. government, with 61.47% of primary care health professional shortage areas (HPSAs) located in rural areas (RHIhub, 2021). In 2019, it was estimated that 80% of rural Americans were medically underserved (Mainder, 2019). This is due to a limited number of healthcare providers: Although 20% of the U.S. population lives in rural areas, only 10% of the nation's physicians practice in rural areas. Rural physicians are typically three years older than their urban counterparts, contributing to an estimated 23% decrease in the number of rural doctors over the next 10 years due to retirement (Mainder, 2019).

Rural workforce shortages before and during the pandemic extended past nursing to include support staff, providers, and administration. HPSAs are determined through the HPSA ratings calculated by the National Health

Service Corps (NHSC) in order to determine priorities for clinician assignments. HPSA scores are calculated for three areas: primary care, mental health, and dental (Figures 3.1–3.3). The score for primary care includes four areas: the population-to-provider ratio (10 points), percentage of the population below 100% of the federal poverty level (5 points), infant health index based on infant mortality rate or low birth weight rate (5 points), and travel time to the source of care outside of the HSPA designation area (5 points).

Dental health HPSA scoring ranges from 0 to 26. The score is also based on four criteria, which include the population-to-provider ratio (10 points), percentage of population below 100% of the federal poverty level (10 points), water fluoridation status (1 point), and travel time to nearest source of care outside of the HPSA designation area (5 points).

Mental health HPSA scoring ranges from 0 to 25. The criteria included to determine the score include the population-to-provider ratio (7 points), percent of population below 100% of the federal poverty level (15 points), elderly (people older than age 65) ratio (3 points), youth (percentage of people younger than age 18) ratio (3 points), alcohol abuse prevalence (1 point), substance abuse prevalence (1 point), and travel to the nearest source of care outside the HPSA designation area (5 points).

HPSA scores are used to determine the need for healthcare providers. A higher HPSA score in any of the three areas discussed earlier translates into a greater need for providers. Providers working in high-HPSA–scored areas can take advantage of educational funding through the NHSC and the Nurses Corps Scholarship and Nurse Corps Loan Repayment programs. Rural critical access hospitals (CAHs) would benefit from using this opportunity for recruitment.

Rural Nurse Practitioners in Clinical Settings

Multiple barriers exist to recruiting primary care providers in rural communities, including advanced practice registered nurses (APRNs). The proposal to address healthcare provider shortages with expanding the APRN's role and responsibilities has been shown to be effective. However, barriers for recruitment include understanding rural communities' low salaries, a lack of adequate office space, limited networks for peer activities, and practice restrictions in areas where APRN practice is restricted from these professionals' full scope of practice due to state laws and policies. Wei et al. (2018) identified recruitment strategies for APRNs, including improvements in work environments, professional autonomy, variety in professional opportunities, and ongoing mental health support to deal with job stress and peer feedback. However, the complications associated with the COVID-19 pandemic eroded the availability of these supports and left APRNs to manage these challenges in professional isolation. To lessen this gap in care, the University of San Francisco offers an APRN major, collaborating with medically underserved rural areas, community-based rural clinics, and rural health departments to lessen this shortage of diverse health providers while simultaneously providing their APRN students with options for clinical rotations and education.

To increase the number of primary care nurse practitioners, clinical nurse specialists, and certified nurse midwives in rural and underserved areas, the Health Resources and Services Administration (HRSA) now offers the Advanced Nursing Education Workforce (ANEW) program. Now in its second cycle, the program's focus is on increasing the number of APRNs who can provide primary care services, mental health and substance use disorder care, and maternal health care (HRSA, 2023). The ANEW program grant offers tuition support to graduate nursing students who commit to serving rural and underserved areas after graduation.

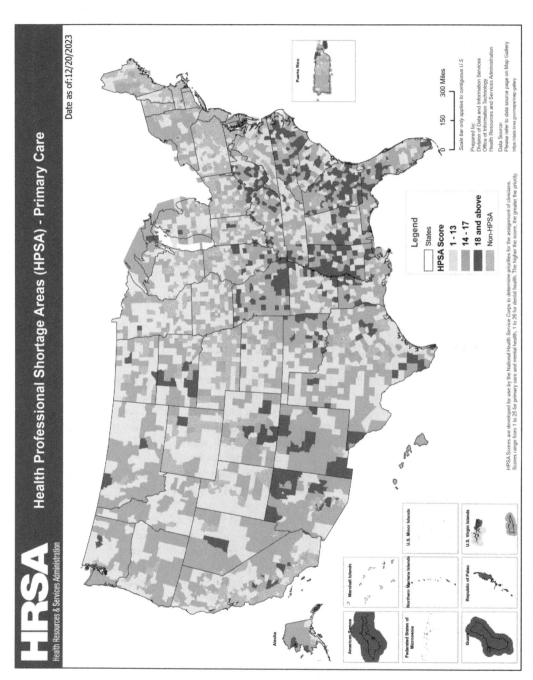

FIGURE 3.1 Health Professional Shortage Areas—Primary Care

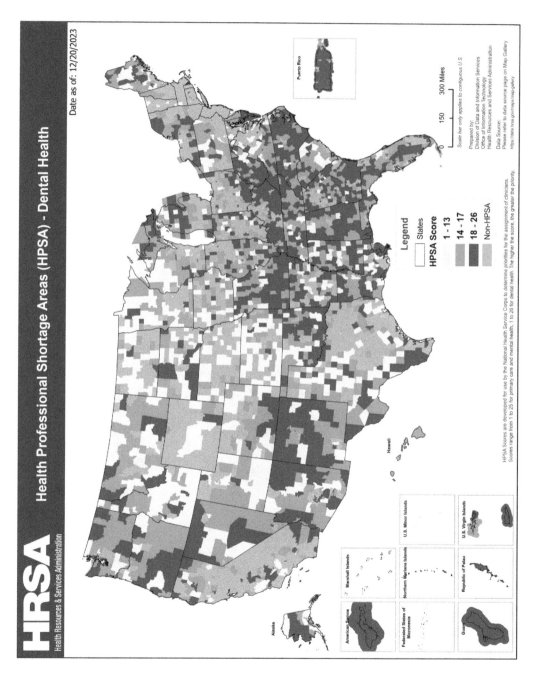

FIGURE 3.2 Health Professional Shortage Areas—Dental Health

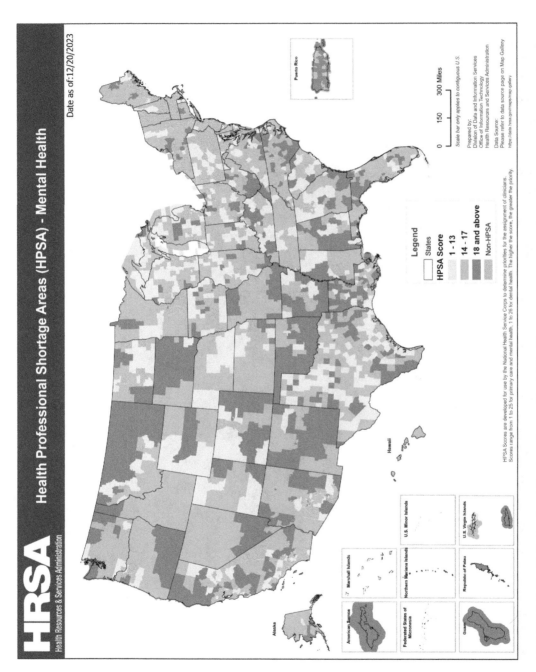

FIGURE 3.3 Health Professional Shortage Areas—Mental Health

Thomas et al. (2021) emphasizes that rural communities often still do not have opportunities to establish care relationships with role models and providers who mirror their race, ethnicity, or culture. Many rural residents do not speak English, and many come from culturally diverse backgrounds that differ from those of their providers. This research aimed to focus on rural primary healthcare needs by creating a clinical immersion that would recruit, train, educate, and evaluate APRN students who had been approved from a rural residency and practice in rural counties. Participants participated in face-to-face interviews to qualify for this 16-week immersion in rural communities. Qualitative data were collected during interviews and feedback sessions. The researchers simultaneously collected quantitative data on process and outcome measures focused on the learning objectives developed for the didactic and clinical portions of the immersion experiences. Data analyses and evaluations were completed to measure the effectiveness of program goals, outcomes, and sustainability and possible expansion of the program.

Thomas et al. (2021) reported that this project contributed to success for both APRN students and their preceptors for a four-year period. The researchers attributed this success to several factors, including:

1. Adherence to in-person interviews
2. An extensive orientation, one that lasted for at least a full day in the rural community; it was noted to be more helpful than any online education or review of the literature
3. A weekly debriefing of APRN students with the program manager who completed either weekly rural visits to each rural clinic to resolve programmatic issues and those related to housing or a weekend community outreach program
4. Positive relationships and collaborations with clinical partners and community stakeholders

"Rural communities often overlooked and invisible are now becoming part of the fabric of graduate education in an urban university serving minorities" (Thomas et al., p. 58).

A clinical environment that motivates staff and supports a sense of belonging can be particularly challenging in rural settings in which staffing is often at a minimum, and geographic boundaries, weather, and technology may add to feelings of disconnectedness or lack of belonging. These added stressors in rural and remote areas put newly graduated registered nurses at a higher risk for transition shock and may fuel their decision to leave their workplace setting or the profession entirely. Van Rooyen et al. (2018) attempted to examine and describe available practice guidelines that focus on the transition of final-year nursing students into the role of professional nurses. The researchers designed the following five-step integrative process to ease the transition to advanced practice and promote retention in rural settings:

Step 1: Formulation of the review question: The investigators sought to answer the question, What are the best available guidelines to develop a best-practice guideline (BPG) for transitioning senior nursing students to professional nurses?

Step 2: Review of the literature: The investigators conducted a systematic review of the literature with the assistance of an experienced research librarian. The initial search was completed in 2014 and updated in 2017. BPGs based on systematic reviews and on guidelines regarding transitions to practice were included in the study. Research published between 2008 and 2017 was included; however, literature on transitions relating to other healthcare professionals was excluded from the study.

Step 3: Data analysis: Data from eight practice guidelines resulted in the emergence of three themes that supported the transition of the final year of nursing students to professional nurses. The themes identified were as follows:

- Support is needed for final-year nursing students and new graduates
- There exists the need for socialization and belonging
- A positive clinical learning environment is required

Step 4: Thematic data analysis: This analysis allowed the researchers to examine the research topic thoughtfully and systematically to best evaluate its trustworthiness, value, and currency in a particular context, one considering the qualitative paradigm of the guidelines (van Rooyen et al., 2018).

Step 5: Scoping review: The researchers used a complete search and selection process to extract BPGs from the remaining raw data and consider them for inclusion. Data from each guideline were evaluated using the AGREE II (Appraisal of Guidelines for Research and Evaluation II) instrument. Data appraisal, extraction, and synthesis were conducted by the third and fourth authors of the study, who assumed roles as independent appraisers to support the study's trustworthiness.

The three themes that emerged from the review of eight BPGs are interconnected and equally essential to facilitating the transition of nursing students and newly graduated registered nurses into nursing practice. According to van Rooyen et al. (2018), socialization and belonging can be encouraged to support students and new graduates, fostering a positive learning environment. Socialization instills feelings of belonging, which enhances confidence and the acceptance of responsibility and accountability for delivering safe patient care (Zarshenas et al., 2014).

Distance and Transportation

Nearly one-quarter (23%) of rural residents report that access to high-quality providers is a major problem in their communities (Lam et al., 2018). One factor believed to affect these residents is that travel to a hospital takes them longer, in both time and distance. On average, rural residents live 10.5 miles from a hospital, compared with their suburban counterparts at 5.6 miles and their urban counterparts at 4.4 miles (Lam et al., 2018). Not only is the distance longer, but the travel time is also longer for rural residents, at 17 minutes compared with suburban and urban residents at 12 and 10 minutes, respectively (Lam et al., 2018).

Distance affects health care in rural areas for patients and healthcare workers (Figure 3.4). Patients experience challenges when needing to travel to medical appointments and the hospital for care due to lack of transportation, limited funds for fuel, and distant geographic locations. While patients experience difficulties, so do nurses. Nurses may have a vehicle and money for fuel but still be limited by challenging road conditions, particularly during inclement weather.

Broadband Access

Although at one time telehealth (U.S. Department of Health & Human Services, n.d.) was seen as a less-than-effective patient care tool, during the pandemic, it became the preferred

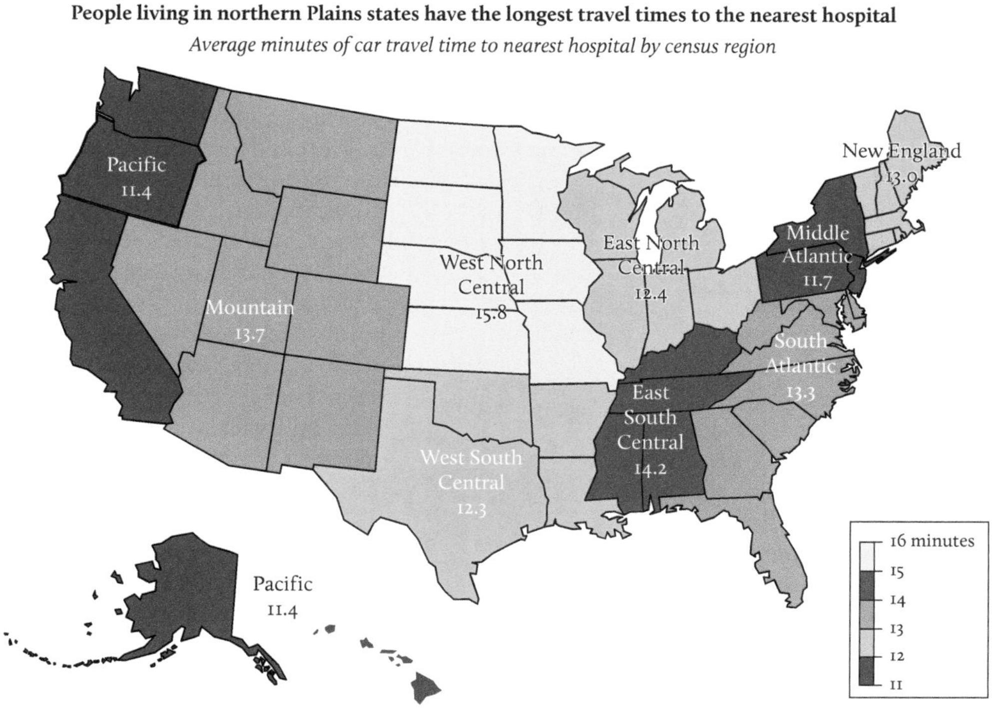

People living in northern Plains states have the longest travel times to the nearest hospital

Average minutes of car travel time to nearest hospital by census region

New England
13.0

Pacific
11.4

Middle
Atlantic
11.7

West North
Central
15.8

East North
Central
12.4

Mountain
13.7

South
Atlantic
13.3

East
South
Central
14.2

West South
Central
12.3

Pacific
11.4

16 minutes
15
14
13
12
11

FIGURE 3.4 Travel Times to Nearest Hospital by Census Region

model for both providers and patients. Prior to the pandemic, reimbursement of telehealth appointments was less than the cost of actual doctor visits. However, recognizing the effectiveness of telehealth, the Centers for Medicare & Medicaid Services quickly changed this to accommodate the continuum of care. Private insurance companies followed, but legislative and other government agencies continue to be reluctant to change even though satisfaction with telehealth visits is high.

Telehealth offers multiple new methods of healthcare delivery. *Telehealth* is defined as the use of technology to support and promote long-distance clinical health care, health education, public health, and health administration through four modalities established by the HRSA:

- Live conferencing
- Storing and forwarding
- Remote patient monitoring
- Mobile health

Telehealth can increase access to preventative and specialty care, address health disparities, and reduce healthcare cost (Kearly et al., 2020). In rural and underserved areas, it can help address transportation barriers and healthcare provider shortages. However, expanding telehealth to rural and underserved areas comes with challenges. To expand telehealth successfully across state and territorial agencies, three key needs have been identified (Kearly et al., 2020). First, states or areas need to have adequate telehealth infrastructure, including broadband access and telehealth networks. Second, there must be collaboration between the states, regions, state government agencies, and partnerships working to overcome telehealth challenges. Third, there must be coordination to reform public and commercial telehealth policies (Kearly et al., 2020).

Funding and reimbursement are barriers to telehealth. "As of 2019, 50 states and the District of Columbia reimburse for live video through their Medicaid programs, whereas only 21 reimburse for remote patient monitoring and 11 reimburse for store and forward" (Kearly et al., 2020, p. 89). From the start of the pandemic in 2020, patient monitoring claims to Medicare and private insurance companies grew four times in one year (Tang et al., 2022). Some states and territorial areas have developed funding opportunities and/or contracts that include telehealth and the development of training opportunities for providers via telehealth and Project ECHO.

Unfortunately, many rural hospitals are already budget-strapped, which limits their ability to remain current with technological trends, including innovative technology and telehealth (Mosley et al., 2020). Because of the older population in rural settings, many patients may have a lack of trust in the services offered through telehealth and believe they might result in a compromise of their privacy as the provider on the other end of the visit is not known to the patient. Many rural CAHs took advantage of federal fiscal support such as the Coronavirus Aid, Relief, and Economic Security (CARES) Act to bolster their telehealth capacity and worked to improve interactions between providers and patients, with trending success. Increased use of telehealth was seen highest in disadvantaged populations (Weil, 2022). According to the Federal Communications Commission (FCC), 22.3% of rural residents and 27.7% of Americans living on tribal land lack broadband coverage when compared with only 1.5% of urban residents. To address this disparity, the Rural Development Broadband ReConnect Program was developed. The ReConnect Loan and Grant program provided funds for construction, improvement, and acquisition of facilities and equipment to provide broadband services (U.S. Department of Agriculture, 2022). The federal government has also been working to increase broadband access through the American Broadband Initiative, which details the strategy to identify and remove barriers to broadband access and expand the U.S. broadband infrastructure (National Telecommunications and Information Administration, 2022).

Although the telehealth capability addresses provider issues, it does not always improve access to health care as many rural residents do not have broadband access and thus do not have the ability to see an actual provider, contributing to poorer health outcomes. The FCC (2023) mapped broadband health in America in 2017 to determine areas of the United States where broadband access is limited. To offer current information related to broadband access, both urban and rural, the FCC developed a website that provides an overview of broadband availability in the United States (Figure 3.5). The website allows users to filter rural information by percentage of rural population and health measure. The website can be accessed at https://www.fcc.gov/reports-research/maps/connect2health/index.html#ll=40,-95&z=4&t=insights&inb=in_bb_access&inh=in_diabetes_rate&dm-f=none&inc=none&slb=90,100&slh=10,22

Health Insurance Coverage

Many rural residents are uninsured or underinsured, which leads to a limited number of treatments based on expenses. Adding to their limited insurance coverage, many rural residents work at jobs at which they cannot afford to take a day off to seek treatment. The COVID-19 pandemic has had a large impact on insurance coverage. During the pandemic, many individuals lost their jobs, which resulted in a loss of insurance coverage. Before the implementation of the Affordable Care Act (ACA) (HealthCare.gov, n.d.), individuals who lost their job had limited health insurance options (Agarwal & Sommers, 2020). The ACA created several new health insurance options for rural residents who lose their health insurance due

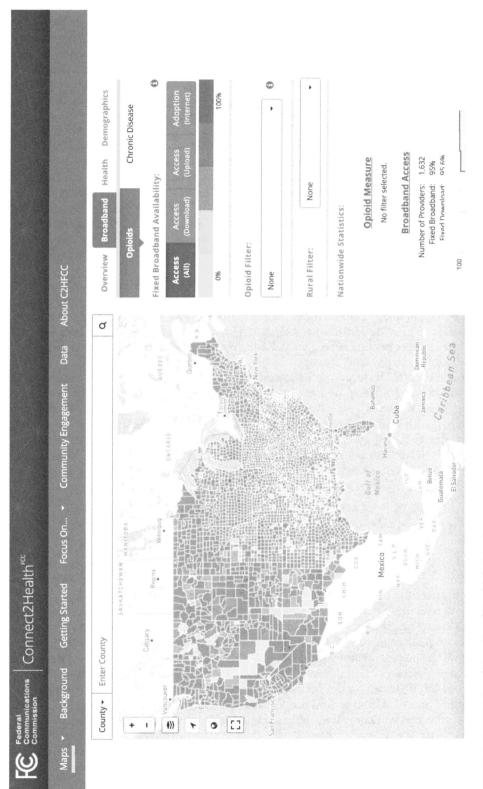

FIGURE 3.5 FCC Map of Broadband Health in America

to unemployment, especially that which is related to the pandemic. Opportunities for health insurance were increased in the 36 states that opted to expand their Medicaid programs by removing categorical eligibility requirements, extending eligibility to all U.S. citizens, and qualifying documented immigrants with incomes below the 138% of the federal poverty level (Agarwal & Sommers, 2020). Hispanic and Black workers suffered job loss at greater percentages during the pandemic, which reduced the ACA's potential to protect against becoming uninsured by 7.0 percentage points and 13.9 percentage points, respectively (Agarwal & Sommers, 2020). Other persistent gaps include a lack of coverage options for undocumented immigrants, who are ineligible for public programs or marketplace subsidies.

Although there is access to affordable care in rural America, challenges also exist. Medicaid and the Healthcare Marketplace offer sources of affordable healthcare coverage for rural residents, with the American Rescue Plan (The White House, 2021) strengthening rural options. Access to these programs has resulted in a decrease in the number of uninsured residents in rural areas. However, challenges to health care in rural areas extend past healthcare coverage; a lack of access to care remains in many areas due to provider shortages, infrastructure limitations, and long distances to care (Assistant Secretary for Planning and Evaluation [ASPE], 2021).

In addition to supporting the development of primary care providers in rural areas, the Department of Health and Human Services offered grants to healthcare clinics and centers to support rural primary care facilities. One example is HRSA's funding of community health centers to provide community-based care and culturally competent primary and specialty care. These centers served vulnerable populations, providing care regardless of individuals' ability to pay (ASPE, 2021).

The Rural Health Clinic program affected access to care for rural residents. Healthcare facilities that met certain requirements were reimbursed at enhanced Medicare and Medicaid rates. These facilities were located in rural underserved areas that meet the necessary requirements, such as using a team approach to delivering care, with physicians working with nurse practitioners and physician assistants. While these clinics offer an avenue to health care for rural residents, they are not required to provide care regardless of insurance status or an individual's ability to pay (ASPE, 2021).

Conclusion

Access to healthcare services in rural areas continues to be limited. There have been workforce shortages in rural areas over the past few decades with projections that the shortages will not improve. To ensure all rural residents receive the healthcare services they deserve, there must be many changes made to rural healthcare delivery. The NHSC has been successful at placing healthcare providers in U.S. rural and underserved areas; however, many providers complete their service commitment and then move to another practice. Due to this fact and the increasing number of aging healthcare providers, it is projected there will continue to be shortages in rural areas. This shortage includes nurses. During the pandemic, many nurses left bedside practice and were replaced by traveling nurses who were given a higher rate of pay. Also, many rural nurses who left their positions returned to the same settings as travelers working alongside colleagues at hourly rates that doubled or tripled their former rate of pay. With limited services and the closure of healthcare facilities, rural residents now need to travel farther to seek care. This has led to a hardship for many as they lack the resources to pay for a car, car maintenance, and fuel. An alternative is telehealth, which has been well received and utilized in some rural communities; however, it also has its limitations due to the lack of rural infrastructure to accommodate broadband access.

Eric is the chief executive officer of a CAH in northern Maine. The hospital has been working hard to recruit healthcare providers to its community. To recruit providers, it added the facility to the NHSC list. The hospital had some interest from individuals looking for loan repayment; however, it has not been able to secure providers. Although it has had some providers with a rural background interested in taking a position there, they either were from a rural community or completed some of their clinical hours in a rural setting. Last month, Eric was excited as he had a provider who was interested in working at the hospital. He had worked one on one with the provider to ensure everything went well and that they could secure filling the position. After negotiating a contract with the provider, Eric arranged for the provider to meet with the local realtor to tour the community and available homes. Unfortunately, there were no homes available to purchase, but there was a home available for rent. The provider decided to rent a home while he had a home built; however, he wanted to purchase land prior to signing a contract with the hospital. While meeting with the realtor, the provider found out that while there was land for sale, it could not be developed due to limited infrastructure. The realtor explained how the town had been working on housing with community members and the Chamber of Commerce to figure out how to solve the housing problem; however, all they were able to accomplish was a lot of talking. The provider decided to decline the position, which left the hospital with limited providers once again.

Programs and services such as telehealth, community health clinics, and healthcare workforce programs have helped improve access to health care to rural Americans.

Questions for Discussion Related to Case Study 3.1

1. Discuss potential strategies by which rural healthcare organizations can partner with local governments to ameliorate barriers posed by the housing shortage. Should these organizations receive tax credits if they contribute to strengthening the housing market and infrastructure of rural communities?
2. Is the NHSC supporting the needs of rural healthcare organizations? Should a special commission be formed to examine the NHSC's effectiveness and propose methodologies to expand its reach and resources so that it contributes to the recruitment of staff?

References

Agarwal, S. D., & Sommers, B. D. (2020). Insurance coverage after job loss—The importance of the ACA during the COVID-associated recession. *New England Journal of Medicine, 383*(17), 1603–1606.

Assistant Secretary for Planning and Evaluation. (2021, July 9). *Access to affordable care in rural America: Current trends and key challenges.* https://aspe.hhs.gov/sites/default/files/2021-07/rural-health-rr.pdf

Council on Graduate Medical Education. (2020). *Rural health policy brief 1.* https://www.hrsa.gov/sites/default/files/hrsa/advisory-committees/graduate-medical-edu/publications/cogme-rural-health-policy-brief.pdf

Federal Communications Commission. (2022). *Connect2Health: Mapping broadband health in America 2017*. https://www.fcc.gov/reports-research/maps/connect2health/index.html#ll=40,-95&z=4&t=insights&inb=in_bb_rural_access&inh=in_diabetes_rate&dmf=none&inc=none&slb=0,100&slh=14,22

HealthCare.gov. (n.d.). *Affordable Care Act (ACA)*. https://www.healthcare.gov/glossary/affordable-care-act/

Health Resources and Services Administration. (2023). *Advanced Nursing Education Workforce (ANEW) program*. https://www.hrsa.gov/grants/find-funding/HRSA-23-014

Janke, A. T., Mei, H., Rothenberg, C., Becher, R. D., Len, Z., & Venkatesh, A. (2021). Analysis of hospital resource availability and COVID-19 mortality across the United States. *Journal of Hospital Medicine, 16*(4), 211–214.

Kearly, A., Oputa, J., & Harper-Hardy, P. (2020). Health agencies to improve access to needed health services. *Journal of Public Health Management & Practice, 26*(1), 86–90.

Lam, O., Broderick, B., & Toor, S. (2018). *How far Americans live from the closest hospital differs by community type*. Pew Research Center. https://www.pewresearch.org/short-reads/2018/12/12/how-far-americans-live-from-the-closest-hospital-differs-by-community-type/

Mainder, V. (2019). *Lack of healthcare access in rural America*. PrognoCIS. https://prognocis.com/lack-of-health-care-access-in-rural-america/

Mosley, D., DeBehnke, D., Gaskell, S., & Weil, A. (2020). *2020 rural hospital sustainability index: trends in rural hospital financial viability, community essentially, and outpatient outmigration*. Navigant. https://guidehouse.com/-/media/www/site/ insights/healthcare/2019/navigant-rural-hospital- analysis-22019.pdf

National Telecommunications and Information Administration. (2022). *American Broadband Initiative: Progress report*. https://www.ntia.doc.gov/report/2020/ABI_Progress_Report

Rural Health Information Hub. (2022). *Healthcare access in rural communities*. https://www.ruralhealthinfo.org/topics/healthcare-access

Tang, M., Mehrotra, A., & Stern, A. D. (2022). Rapid growth of remote patient monitoring is driven by a small number of primary care providers. *Health Affairs, 41*(9), 1248–1254. https://doi.org/10.1377/hlthaff.2021.02026

The White House. (2021, January 20). *President Biden announces American Rescue Plan*. https://www.whitehouse.gov/briefing-room/legislation/2021/01/20/president-biden-announces-american-rescue-plan/

Thomas, T. I. L., Caldera, M., & Glymph, D. (2021). Collaboration, culture and communication: Preparing the next generation to provide rural primary health care. *Journal of Nursing Education and Practice, 11*(6), 50.

U.S. Department of Agriculture. (2022). *ReConnect Loan and Grant program*. https://www.usda.gov/reconnect

U.S. Department of Health & Human Services. (n.d.). *Telehealth*. https://telehealth.hhs.gov/patients/understanding-telehealth

U.S. Department of Health and Human Services. (n.d.). *Underserved group*. https://toolkit.ncats.nih.gov/glossary/underserved-group/#:~:text=The%20U.S.%20Health%20Services%20Administration,or%20a%20high%20elderly%20population

van Rooyen, D. R. M., Jordan, P. J., ten Ham-Baloyi, W., & Caka, E. M. (2018). A comprehensive literature review of guidelines facilitating transition of newly graduated nurses to professional nurses. *Nurse Education in Practice, 30*, 35–41. https://doi.org/10.1016/j.nepr.2018.02.010

Wei, H., Roberts, P., Strickler, J., & Corbett, R. W. (2019). Nurse leaders' strategies to foster nurse resilience. *Journal of Nursing Management, 27*(4), 681–687. https://doi.org/10.1111/jonm.12736

Weil, A. R. (2022). Telemedicine, disparities, pharmaceuticals, and more. *Health Affairs, 41*(5), 621. https://doi.org/10.1377/hlthaff.2022.00449

Zarshenas, L., Sharif, F., Molazem, Z., Khayyer, M., Zare, N., & Ebadi, E. (2014). Professional socialization in nursing: A qualitative content analysis. *Iran Journal of Nurse Midwifery Research*, *19*(4), 423–438.

Image Credits

CHAPTER 4

Access to Acute Services

Many rural hospitals were built in the post–World War II era. Since then, the level of care and number of patients have changed, resulting in a decrease in patient volume. As a result, many rural hospitals are overstaffed and underused. The average rural hospital has 25 beds and an average daily census of seven patients (Wishner et al., 2016). As a result, staffing ratios are different in rural hospitals from those in urban facilities. During the COVID-19 pandemic, healthcare access in rural America became even more limited, which affected the financial solvency of many healthcare facilities, especially in rural areas. In an attempt to limit the spread of COVID-19, many hospitals increased their inpatient capability while decreasing or closing their outpatient departments and postponing or canceling elective visits and procedures (Khullar et al., 2020). However, elective procedures provide a greater income for many rural facilities. In 2014, the Agency for Healthcare Research and Quality estimated that elective admissions accounted for more than 30% of total inpatient revenue, with hospitals earning $700 more for an elective admission than from an admission through the emergency department (ED; Khullar et al., 2020). Some hospitals experienced a loss in revenue due to state and federal guidance requesting the minimization of nonessential services (Khullar et al., 2020).

Over the past decade, there has been an increase in rural hospital closures, and many rural facilities are at risk of closing (Table 4.1; Suttle, 2019). At the beginning of 2023, multiple hospitals across the United States were at risk of closing due to inadequate reimbursements (Robertson, 2023). Table 4.2 demonstrates a list of the hospitals with a three-year margin of -10% or greater based on data from the Centers for Medicare & Medicaid Services (CMS). Data from 2020 were excluded due to unusual cost and revenue changes from the pandemic (Robertson, 2023). Although this table demonstrates the number of hospitals that are at risk of closing, it does not depict the number of hospitals that have closed over the past few decades. Table 4.3 presents the number of hospitals that have closed and that are at risk for closing per state (Center for Healthcare Quality and Payment Reform [CHQPR], 2023).

TABLE 4.1 Hospitals at High Risk of Closure

State	Rural Hospitals at High Risk	Percentage of Rural Hospitals at High Risk
Tennessee	19	68%
Alabama	18	60%
Oklahoma	28	60%
Arkansas	18	53%
Mississippi	25	50%
West Virginia	9	50%
South Carolina	4	44%
Georgia	14	41%
Kentucky	18	40%
Louisiana	11	37%
Kansas	26	31%

Source: Mosley et al. (2020).

TABLE 4.2 Rural Hospitals With the Worst Three-Year Margins

Hospital	Location	Number of Beds	Total 2021 Expense (in Millions)	Three-Year Margin on Patient Services	Three-Year Total Margin
Thomasville Regional Medical Center	Thomasville, Alabama	29	$16.6M	−53.1%	−46.2%
Medical University of South Carolina (MUSC) Health Marion Medical Center	Mullins, South Carolina	124	$46.6M	−24.7	−43.2%
Defiance Regional Medical Center	Defiance, Ohio	35	$87M	36.4%	−39.2%
Lallie Kemp Regional Medical Center	Independence, Louisiana	24	$46.9M	−41.2%	−30.0%
Hill Regional Hospital	Hillsboro, Texas	25	$28.8M	−2.1%	−34.8%
Stroud Regional Medical Center	Stroud, Oklahoma	25	$57.5M	−31.7%	−33.4%

TABLE 4.2 Rural Hospitals With the Worst Three-Year Margins (*Continued*)

Hospital	Location	Number of Beds	Total 2021 Expense (in Millions)	Three-Year Margin on Patient Services	Three-Year Total Margin
Big Sky Medical Center	Big Sky, Montana	4	$16.7M	−28.3%	−31.7%
The Physician's Hospital in Anadarko	Anadarko, Oklahoma	25	$68M	−29.7%	−31.2%
Ascension Saint Thomas Stones River	Woodbury, Tennessee	55	$11.4M	−36.4%	−30.8%
Fairfax Community Hospital	Fairfax, Oklahoma	25	$32.7M	−38.5%	−29.6%
Bon Secours—Southern Virginia Regional Medical Center	Emporia, Virginia	80	$28.6M	−10.1%	−29.4%
Westfield Memorial Hospital	Westfield, New York	4	$11.7M	−38.1%	−29.1%
Baptist Health Fishermen's Community Hospital	Marathon, Florida	8	$25.7M	−29.2%	−29.0%
CHI St. Joseph Health Bellville Hospital	Bellville, Texas	32	$16.7M	−40.4%	−28.2%
Ascension Sacred Heart Hospital Gulf	Port Saint Joe, Florida	19	$23.5M	−31.1%	−27.1%
Fostoria Community Hospital	Fostoria, Ohio	15	$45.9M	22.7%	−26.9%
Ascension Saint Thomas DeKalb Hospital	Smithville, Texas	71	$14.1M	−26.5%	−26.6%
Lanai Community Hospital	Lanai City, Hawaii	4	$6.2M	−25.7%	−23.7%
Ascension Seton Smithville Hospital	Smithville, Texas	36	$16.1M	−25.7%	−23.7%
Pineville Community Health Center	Pineville, Kentucky	120	$13.8M	−46.5%	−23.0%
Stillwater Medical—Perry	Perry, Oklahoma	26	$9.7M	−32.2%	−22.8%

(continued)

TABLE 4.2 Rural Hospitals With the Worst Three-Year Margins (*Continued*)

Hospital	Location	Number of Beds	Total 2021 Expense (in Millions)	Three-Year Margin on Patient Services	Three-Year Total Margin
Izard County Medical Center	Calico Rock, Arkansas	25	$7.1M	−28.7%	−21.8%
Big South Fork Medical Center	Oneida, Tennessee	25	$11.8M	−19.8%	−21.5%
Unicoi County Hospital	Erwin, Tennessee	10	$11.1M	−21.4%	−20.9%
Bob Wilson Memorial Hospital	Ulysses, Kansas	45	$13.6M	−34.3%	−20.5%
Bon Secours—Southampton Memorial Hospital	Franklin, Virginia	221	$57.9M	−3.9%	−20.4%
Eureka Springs Hospital Commission	Eureka Springs, Arkansas	15	$8.2M	−23.4%	−20.1%
Haskell Regional Hospital	Stigler, Oklahoma	25	$10.1M	−23.1%	−19.8%
Vanderbilt Bedford Hospital	Shelbyville, Tennessee	104	$37.5M	−2.9%	−19.4%
Highland Community Hospital	Picayune, Mississippi	60	$53.3M	−12.8%	−18.2%
Carilion Tazewell Community Hospital	Tazewell, Virginia	238	$19.6M	− 4.3%	−18.2%
Colusa Medical Center	Colusa, California	48	$29.8M	−9.4%	−18.1%
Rush County Memorial Hospital	LaCrosse, Kansas	24	$7.6M	−27.4%	−18.1%
Kiowa County Memorial Hospital	Greensbury, Kansas	25	$9.9M	−30.6%	−18.0%
Mercyhealth Hospital and Medical Center—Walworth	Lake Geneva, Wisconsin	25	$558.7M	433.9%	=17.9%
Muscogee (Creek) Nation Medical Center	Okmulgee, Oklahoma	20	$28.4M	−35.4%	−17.8%
Hillsboro Community Hospital	Hillsboro, Kansas	15	$9.3M	−32.3%	−17.7%

TABLE 4.2 Rural Hospitals With the Worst Three-Year Margins (*Continued*)

Hospital	Location	Number of Beds	Total 2021 Expense (in Millions)	Three-Year Margin on Patient Services	Three-Year Total Margin
MUSC Health Lancaster Medical Center	Lancaster, South Carolina	217	$111M	−8.4%	−17.1%
Glenn Medical Center	Willows, California	47	$33.6M	−18.6%	−16.8%
Sparrow Carson Hospital	Carson City, Michigan	87	$50.3M	−9.6%	−16.8%
Washington County Hospital Inc.	Plymouth, North Carolina	25	$20.8M	−17.2%	−16.6%
Creek Nation Community Hospital	Okemah, Oklahoma	25	$19.4M	−64.0%	−16.6%
Sanford Aberdeen Medical Center	Aberdeen, South Dakota	48	$76.4M	−24.5%	−15.7%
MidCoast Medical Center—Central	Llano, Texas	25	$7M	−6.4%	−15.7%
Sharon Hospital	Sharon, Connecticut	78	$65.1M	−13.4%	−15.6%
Hillcrest Hospital Cushing	Cushing, Oklahoma	99	$16.4M	2.2%	=15.2%
Crosbyton Clinic Hospital	Crosbyton, Texas	2	$4.6M	−42.5%	−15.1%
Kau Hospital	Pahala, Hawaii	21	$30.2M	−34.8%	−14.9%
Tanner Medical Center/East Alabama	Wedowee, Alabama	15	$13.7M	−40.6%	−14.8%
Atrium Health Floyd Cherokee Medical Center	Centre, Alabama	60	$15.3M	−16.7%	−14.8%
McKenzie County Healthcare Systems Inc.	Watford City, North Dakota	24	$45.8M	−22.7%	−14.5%
Gundersen St. Elizabeth's Hospital and Clinics	Wabasha, Minnesota	25	$44.3M	−19.6%	−14.5%

(*continued*)

TABLE 4.2 Rural Hospitals With the Worst Three-Year Margins (*Continued*)

Hospital	Location	Number of Beds	Total 2021 Expense (in Millions)	Three-Year Margin on Patient Services	Three-Year Total Margin
AllianceHealth Madill	Madill, Texas	25	$16.5M	−13.2%	−14.5%
University of Pittsburgh Medical Center (UPMC) Lock Haven	Lock Haven, Pennsylvania	25	$42.1M	−14.1%	−14.4%
MUSC Health Chester Medical Center	Chester, South Carolina	82	$53.2M	−12.5%	−14.3%
North Baldwin Infirmary	Bay Minette, Alabama	78	$45.9M	−8.3%	−14.2%
Ascension St. Thomas Highlands Hospital	Sparta, Tennessee	60	$22.2M	−18.6%	−14.1%
Margaretville Memorial Hospital	Margaretville, New York	15	$25.1M	−23.6%	−13.7%
Helena Regional Medical Center	Helena, Arkansas	155	$23.4M	−12.9%	−13.6%
Carle Richland Memorial Hospital	Olney, Illinois	123	$65.6M	1.2%	−13.2%
Baptist Memorial Hospital—Carroll County	Huntingdon, Tennessee	70	$26.3M	−13.1%	−13.2%
Lakeland Community Hospital	Haleyville, Alabama	49	$23.1M	−9.9%	−13.1%
Fillmore Community Hospital	Fillmore, Utah	19	$10.5M	3.6%	−13.0%
UPMC Jameson	New Castle, Pennsylvania	123	$122.4M	−6.4%	−12.9%
PeaceHealth Ketchikan Medical Center	Ketchikan, Arkansas	25	$94.7M	−3.1%	−12.6%
McLaren Central Michigan	Mount Pleasant, Michigan	151	$147.2M	−14.4%	−15.5%
Marion Regional Medical Center	Hamilton, Alabama	57	$22.5M	−18.7%	−12.1%

TABLE 4.2 Rural Hospitals With the Worst Three-Year Margins (*Continued*)

Hospital	Location	Number of Beds	Total 2021 Expense (in Millions)	Three-Year Margin on Patient Services	Three-Year Total Margin
UPMC Horizon	Greenville, Pennsylvania	157	$151.2M	−2.3%	−12.1%
Lee County Community Hospital	Pennington Gap, Virginia	6	$20.6M	−1.7%	−12.0%
Franciscan Health Rensselaer	Rensselaer, Indiana	25	$35.9M	−6.9%	−11.7%
Alliance Health-care System, Inc.	Holly Springs, Mississippi	40	$12.2M	−11.5%	−11.7%
Community Memorial Hospital	Hicksville, Ohio	25	$34.3M	−10.4%	−11.7%
Haskell Memorial Hospital	Haskell, Texas	25	$13.8M	−34.2%	−11.7%
Carnegie Tri-County Municipal Hospital	Carnegie, Oklahoma	21	$19.2M	−15.1%	−11.6%
Providence Sea-side Hospital	Seaside, Oregon	25	$83.5M	1.4%	−11.6%
Monument Health Custer Hospital	Custer, South Dakota	11	$29.4M	−14.4%	−11.5%
UCHealth Pikes Peak Regional Hospital	Woodland Park, Colorado	15	$26.6M	−8.0%	−11.4%
Aspirus Merrill Hospital	Merrill, Wisconsin	25	$20.7M	−0.2%	−11.4%
SGMC Health—Lanier	Lakeland, Georgia	25	$18.8M	−17.1%	−11.0%
Geary Community Hospital	Junction City, Kansas	92	$42.7M	−22.2%	−11.0%
UPMC Chautauqua	Jamestown, New York	88	$131.7M	−17.9%	−11.0%
Hancock County Hospital	Sneedville, Tennessee	10	$7.2M	−6.7%	−11.0%
Johnson County Community Hospital	Mountain City, Tennessee	2	$9.2M	−11.5%	−10.9%

(*continued*)

TABLE 4.2 Rural Hospitals With the Worst Three-Year Margins (*Continued*)

Hospital	Location	Number of Beds	Total 2021 Expense (in Millions)	Three-Year Margin on Patient Services	Three-Year Total Margin
Patients Choice Medical Center of Smith County	Raleigh, Mississippi	29	$2.9M	4.8%	−10.7%
Providence St. Joseph's Hospital	Chewelah, Washington	17	$20.4M	−0.2%	−10.7%
Crenshaw Community Hospital	Luverne, Alabama	65	$15M	−22.6%	−10.6%
Falls Community Hospital and Clinic	Marlin, Texas	44	$12.7M	−24.2%	−10.6%
Martin General Hospital	Williamston, North Carolina	49	$27.7M	−7/1%	−10.5%
Randolph Hospital	Asheboro, North Carolina	145	$114M	−72%	−10.5%
Rappahannock General Hospital	Kilmarnock, Virginia	35	$40.5M	−14.5%	−10.5%
Othello Community Hospital	Othello, Washington	16	$20.5M	−19.0%	−10.5%
Mangum Regional Medical Center	Mangum, Oklahoma	18	$16.7M	−15.8%	−10.3%
Prisma Health Oconee Memorial Hospital	Seneca, South Carolina	169	$188.1M	−7.0%	−10.3%
Platte County Memorial Hospital	Wheatland, Wyoming	25	$25.5M	−8.4%	−10.3%
Marion General Hospital	Columbia, Mississippi	79	$16.5M	−17.2%	−10.2%
Scenic Mountain Medical Center	Big Spring, Texas	132	$45.9M	−9.4%	−10.1%
Bronson South Haven Hospital	South Haven, Michigan	82	$37.9M	−18.9%	−10.1%
Kohala Hospital	Kapaau, Hawaii	25	$14.2M	−38.0%	−10.0%

Source: Marcus Robertson, "100 Hospitals with the Worst Margins Nationwide, Ranked," https://www.becker-shospitalreview.com/finance/101-hospitals-with-the-worst-margins-nationwide-ranked.html. Copyright © 2023 by Becker's Healthcare.

Data were determined by subtracting cumulative costs from cumulative revenues over the given period and then dividing the result by the same cumulative cost figure. This is different from the standard for-profit business approach of using revenues in the denominator.

TABLE 4.3 Rural Hospitals at Risk of Closing

State	Closures Since 2005	Current Number of Rural Hospitals	Hospitals With Losses on Services[1]	
			Number	Percentage
Kansas	10	102	84	82%
Texas	25	159	101	64%
Oklahoma	10	77	57	74%
Mississippi	6	73	46	63%
New York	6	51	41	80%
Alabama	7	52	34	65%
Tennessee	14	55	22	40%
Georgia	9	68	32	47%
Arkansas	2	49	36	73%
Kentucky	4	72	30	42%
California	9	56	33	59%
Missouri	10	57	30	53%
Iowa	1	93	66	71%
Michigan	3	63	23	37%
Louisiana	2	53	36	68%
Maine	3	25	14	56%
Minnesota	6	95	40	42%
South Carolina	4	23	12	52%
West Virginia	5	28	14	50%
Illinois	5	71	19	27%
Indiana	4	52	13	25%
North Carolina	12	52	18	35%
Pennsylvania	6	41	16	39%
South Dakota	3	48	14	29%
Virginia	2	29	10	34%
Colorado	0	42	16	38%
Florida	8	21	9	43%
Montana	0	55	35	64%
Ohio	2	70	17	24%

(continued)

TABLE 4.3 Rural Hospitals at Risk of Closing (*Continued*)

State	Closures Since 2005	Current Number of Rural Hospitals	Hospitals With Losses on Services[1]	
			Number	Percentage
Alaska	1	17	10	59%
North Dakota	1	39	26	67%
Vermont	0	13	10	77%
Idaho	0	29	15	52%
Nebraska	2	71	28	39%
Nevada	2	13	11	85%
New Mexico	1	27	15	56%
Washington	1	40	26	65%
Arizona	4	27	15	56%
Connecticut	0	3	2	67%
Hawaii	0	12	10	83%
Massachusetts	1	5	3	60%
New Hampshire	0	17	7	41%
Wisconsin	1	75	22	29%
Wyoming	0	23	11	48%
Delaware	0	2	0	0%
Maryland	1	4	0	0%
New Jersey	1	0	0	0%
Oregon	0	32	14	44%
Rhode Island	0	0	0	0%
Utah	0	21	7	33%

[1]*Rural hospitals that had a negative margin (loss) on patient services in the most recent year available.*
Data current as of October 2023.
Source: CHQPR (2023).

Hospital closures reduce access to emergency care. Most visits to rural hospital EDs are urgent care or primary care due to limited community-based care. Federally qualified health centers in or near the community can address primary care needs. In rural areas, EDs serve as a safety net for trauma victims, acute illness, patients with cardiac distress, and individuals with acute mental health or substance use needs; these patients could be stabilized and then transferred as needed. When a hospital closes, there is no longer local access to meet these needs. The tendency of uninsured residents in rural communities is to forgo preventative care and delay treatment until their health conditions worsen, which can be exacerbated by the loss of a local hospital. Decisions by the state to expand Medicaid can increase access to needed care for those who are low-income and uninsured. There is a direct correlation between the number of intensive care unit (ICU) beds and community income populations, making an important impact on the hospital revenues and access to care. The COVID-19 pandemic highlighted the importance of ICU beds in preventing death. Disparities exist among community ICU beds based on the U.S. community's median income level (Kanter et al., 2020). When short-term hospitals and critical access hospitals (CAHs) in all 50 states and Washington, D.C., were evaluated for the number of ICU beds per income level, it was determined that there was a large gap in access to ICU beds. Forty-nine percent of the lowest-income communities had no ICU beds, whereas 3% of the highest-income communities had no ICU beds. Income disparities in the availability of community ICU beds were noted to be more acute in rural areas based on ZIP code (Kanter et al., 2020).

The proximity of a major medical center also affects access to care. Comparing the difference between patient load and providers, rural areas have fewer providers caring for more patients. Rural hospital closures contribute to decreased access to care as well as affecting the supply of physicians in a local healthcare system (Germack et al., 2019). Recommendations to improve access to care to communities in areas not in proximately to a major medical setting during a public health emergency (Administration for Strategic Preparedness & Response, n.d.) include identifying the proximity of disadvantaged communities in advance; assembling a national or regional registry of medical response volunteers to mobilize; and transforming the current system to include cross-hospital certification, privileging, and malpractice coverage (Rodriquez, 2020).

The loss of a hospital has an impact on the rural community. In many of these communities, the hospital is one of the largest employers. This results in healthcare workers needing to travel outside their community for work or to move to another area for employment. Hospital closures also have an impact on recruiting new industries and employers to rural areas as some businesses require as a condition of location within an area that their employees have access to a hospital ED in close proximity.

Rural communities are dependent on their rural hospital not only for care but also for the community's economic viability and development. "When a community loses a hospital, the per capita income falls [by] 4%, and the unemployment rate increases by 1.6%" (Mosley et al., 2020, p. 2). Rural hospitals are highly essential to their communities; in the Eastern United States, 34 states are at risk of losing at least 50% of the hospitals considered highly essential, whereas in the West and South, 16 states have 100% of their hospitals considered highly essential (Table 4.4; Mosley et al., 2020).

The number of rural hospital closures has disproportionally occurred in the South, concentrated in 14 states, and among for-profit hospitals and Medicare-dependent hospitals (U.S. Government Accountability Office, 2018). These were the states that declined to fund the expansion of Medicaid made possible by the Affordable Care Act (ACA) (HealthCare.gov, n.d.) in 2014. There are additional factors contributing to these closures, including changes to rural populations. These populations are aging, with a rise in unemployment related to fewer employers and an evaporation of local industry (e.g., mining, textiles, manufacturing, agriculture), resulting in a decrease in wage earners and a loss of employer-provided health insurance coverage. There are shrinking populations, higher numbers of patients on Medicare and Medicaid, economic challenges in the community, aging facilities, outdated payment and delivery system models, and business decisions by corporate owners and operators who do not live in the community.

Federal funding was appropriated in 1947 when Congress approved the Hill-Burton program, providing monies for the construction of public and nonprofit hospitals in rural America. In 1983, Congress mandated the use of fixed, predetermined reimbursement rates for hospitals due to increases in Medicare hospital spending. Even with this change, there

TABLE 4.4 Highly Essential Rural Hospitals at Risk of Closure

State	Highly Essential At-Risk Rural Hospitals	Percentage of Highly Essential At-Risk Rural Hospitals
Mississippi	25	100%
Tennessee	19	100%
Arkansas	18	100%
Kentucky	18	100%
Louisiana	11	100%
Montana	7	100%
California	6	100%
North Carolina	6	100%
Washington	5	100%
Colorado	4	100%
Idaho	4	100%
Oregon	4	100%
New Mexico	3	100%
Wyoming	3	100%
Florida	2	100%
Arizona	1	100%

Source: Mosley et al. (2020).

were many rural hospital closures in the 1980s and 1990s. In response to these closures, CMS implemented the Medicare Rural Hospital Flexibility Program (Flex Program) of 1997, which authorized inpatient and outpatient services to be paid on a "reasonable cost basis" for CAHs.

Many rural hospitals are classified as CAHs, which requires that they have a certain number of inpatient beds and an emergency room and be eligible for cost-plus reimbursement (Mosley et al., 2020). As mentioned earlier, to be classified as a CAH, the hospital must have no more than 25 inpatient beds and be at least 15 miles by secondary road and 35 miles by primary road from the nearest hospital (Wishner et al., 2016). The Flex Program was effective slowing the number of rural hospital closures until the Great Recession of 2008–2009; however, the number of rural hospital closures have continued (Table 4.5).

Rural hospitals typically have negative margins, which predisposes them to difficulty in covering fixed costs. Multiple factors that exacerbate financial distress include fewer patients seeking inpatient care and across-the-board Medicare payment reductions. Prior to hospital closures, privately insured community residents sought care in newer hospital systems outside the rural community. This weakens the hospitals' payer mix, and they are left with high rates of uninsured patients and patients with public insurance (Medicare and Medicaid), which pays lower reimbursement rates. Decreases in Medicare reimbursement rates exacerbate financial pressure on struggling rural hospitals, especially those with

TABLE 4.5 Rural Hospital Closures 2005–2022

Rural Hospital Closure by Era	
2005–2010	43
2010–2022	139
Closure by Medicare Payment Classification (2005–2022)	
Prospective Payment System	74
Critical Access Hospital	64
Medicare Dependent Hospital	30
Sole Community Hospital	11
Rural Referral Center	2
Closures by Rurality (2005–2022)	
Large rural	69
Small rural	71
Isolated rural	42
Complete or Converted Closures (2005–2022)	
Complete	99
Converted	83

Source: University of North Carolina at Chapel Hill,
Cecil G. Sheps Center for Health Services Research (n.d.).

an older patient population. Medicare cuts from budget appropriations and other federal policies have led to lower reimbursement rates. The Hospital Readmissions Reduction Program reduced payments to inpatient hospitals with high readmission rates resulting in lower Medicare reimbursements for many hospitals.

The Department of Health and Human Services administers payment policies and programs to provide financial support for rural hospitals. This support includes special payments designated for rural hospitals that have met certain criteria to receive higher reimbursements for hospital services than standard Medicare payments. However, despite the increased funding that went to CAHs during the pandemic, including increased reimbursement for telehealth, increased compensation through Provider Relief Fund and the Paycheck Protection Program (PPP; Frieden, 2022), many rural facilities still face uncertain futures.

In 2017, the Rural Emergency Acute Care Hospital (REACH) Act was reintroduced but not voted upon by the appropriate committee. This bipartisan legislation allowed CAHs to transform their delivery model to align with the needs of their community without experiencing financial disincentive of losing cost-plus reimbursement (Mosley et al., 2020). The REACH Act would have offered CAHs the opportunity to rid themselves of excess inpatient beds. In exchange for decreasing their number of inpatient beds, the hospitals would have maintained the ability to move patients to a larger hospital and healthcare system. The REACH Act failed to be passed which led to 168 rural hospitals closing since 2005, 35% still offer outpatient services, urgent care, and emergency services to their community (Mosley et al., 2020).

The COVID-19 pandemic influenced the number of rural hospital closures in other ways. In 2020, the number of rural hospitals shutting down was a record-breaking 20 hospitals (Ellison, 2022). Remaining rural hospitals continue to face many challenges, including low patient volume, heavy reliance on government payers, and financial pressure tied to the COVID-19 pandemic; however, federal aid helped partially offset those challenges in 2021 (Ellison, 2022). This trend continued during the pandemic, with only 24 rural hospitals closing from 2020 to 2022. Many facilities have already spent the federal COVID-19 provider relief funds and PPP loans that supported staffing and supply shortages and lower patient demand as patients deferred care during the pandemic. Rural hospitals needed additional funding to be able to continue to provide care to rural Americans. Rural hospitals lobbied for Congress to delay the scheduled 2% cut in Medicare payments and address the Medicare payment proposal for 2023, which did not address the effects of inflation, labor, or supply cost pressures (Dreher, 2022). In 2024, Medicare and Medicaid rural hospital ambulatory payment classification and adjustments to the wage index increased payments 4.2% (Department of Health and Human Services, 2023). Medicare inpatient prospective payment system rates increased by 3.1% (American Hospital Association, 2023).

CASE STUDY 4.1

The pandemic had an impact on rural residents' access to health care. Oftentimes, a CAH stabilizes patients and then transfers them to a larger facility that is able to provide a higher level of care; however, the pandemic affected the ability to transfer patients due to a lack of bed availability in larger facilities. Abby, the chief executive officer at a CAH in the Midwest, was careful not to make rash decisions during the pandemic. As hers was a small CAH, it had no ICU beds, and due to the lack of bed availability in the larger institutions, it kept patients longer than it normally would have. Generally speaking, it stabilizes patients and then got them to where they needed to be. This put additional pressure on the already limited staff of advanced practice providers and physicians.

Abby's team tried to think of ways in which they could help open up beds in the larger facilities so that a bed could be freed up for a more critical patient. The team participated in a patient exchange system by which patients could be transferred to a hospital that could manage the necessary care. The more severe acute patients were sent to larger healthcare systems, and the stable nonacute patients were sent to the smaller CAHs. This allowed each healthcare facility to function at its highest level of care possible, maximizing the efficiency of both facilities. Abby's team thought that if their hospital could take a recovering skilled care patient from a larger facility, then it would free up a bed, and there would be a bed opening for one of their more advanced acute patients. However, this was not always the case; their hospital, at times, was forced to keep patients longer than it normally would have due to a limited number of beds in acute care hospitals. In addition, the CAH also accepted the recovering COVID-19 patients who were waiting for a bed in a skilled care facility or nursing home. The skilled care facilities and nursing homes had a rule that they could not accept a COVID-19 patient until a certain number of days had passed since they had COVID-19 (due to a CMS regulation). The rural hospitals were able to help by taking the recovering COVID-19 patients as they were not able to go back to their "home" at the nursing home. The CAH ended up keeping patients that it would have normally transferred to a higher-acuity facility due to a limited number of beds. This led to patients dying in their community hospital, which had a large impact on the staff. In just over one month, six community members passed away at the local hospital.

During the pandemic, access to care varied. To offer care to their patients, some hospitals were involved in a patient exchange system by which patients were transferred to a hospital that could manage acute care needs. The acute patients were sent to metropolitan areas, and the stable nonacute patients remained at the rural community hospital. One hospital accepted recovering skill care patients from larger facilities so that the acute care settings had beds available for high-acuity patients in hopes that they would have a bed opening for one of their community members, if needed. This filled an important need for patients who could not transfer from an acute hospital to a skilled care facility as nursing homes had a rule that they would not accept a COVID-19 patient until a certain number of days had passed for the patient to be symptom free. Unfortunately, many times rural CAH hospitals were unable to transfer both acute COVID-19 patients as well as those who would typically have been transferred to a larger tertiary center. This led to many rural residents remaining in the rural CAH, which resulted in higher mortality rates and affecting staff, as receiving the news of a community member's death at another hospital in a larger community is different from caring for the patient in your own facility, where many patients and staff shared commonalities, including family members.

Like all hospitals throughout the country, elective surgeries were canceled for a period of time. In two rural hospitals in the Northwest, the experience was different due to state regulations. One hospital had a period during which it canceled elective surgeries; however, when it was able to resume them, it noted an increase in their number. Another hospital in the Northwest that was not regulated to cancel elective surgeries continued to perform surgeries after a minor interruption and discussion with the surgeons and certified registered nurse anesthetists (CRNAs). Since it was a small hospital with the patient being exposed only to a limited number of staff, it was determined that elective surgeries would continue. This had a positive effect on the hospital's finances as it allowed the facility to care for patients and continue to fill the beds there.

CASE STUDY 4.2

CAHs have a limited number of resources and providers with specialty training. Although the role of CAHs is to stabilize and transfer patients to an acute hospital, they often need assistance with stabilization. To ensure the best care possible for the hospital's community members, the board of directors at a CAH in Iowa purchased the telehealth system E-Hospitalist for the facility's nursing units and emergency room. Having this service ensured that trained physicians were always available. The board believed that E-Hospitalist was the future, as it allowed the hospital to have telemedicine services and support advanced practice providers in the rural setting. It believed that supporting these providers was important due to the physician shortage.

Closure of hospitals and decreases in funding resulted in physicians leaving rural areas to seek alternative positions. Nurses living in rural areas were also forced to seek employment in other locations, requiring commutes and time away from home. With a smaller number of healthcare professionals in the community, the disparities between rural and urban health outcomes become even greater. To compensate for the limited number of trained providers, many rural hospitals have implemented telehealth service. One hospital in the Northwest uses E-Hospitalist on its nursing floor and in the emergency room, where trained physicians are available to support advanced practice providers in the rural setting. Many CAHs believed this was a good addition for the provision of patient care. With the predicted shortage of physicians in rural and remote settings, this type of service supports potential answers for care, giving support to advanced practice registered nurses (APRNs) and physician assistants who are willing to settle in a small community.

Hospital closures have not affected the average annual supply of nurse practitioners (NPs) or CRNAs. From 2010 to 2017, 138 rural counties experienced at least one hospital closure, with 13 counties experiencing two closures (Germack et al., 2021). The counties that experienced hospital closings had a greater percentage of their population living below the federal poverty level (Germack et al., 2021). They also had a greater NP-to-population ratio, demonstrating that NPs have stepped into providing primary care for rural, underserved residents. The NP workforce has been a solution to meeting the nation's primary care needs, especially in rural areas. From 2010 to 2017, the NP workforce grew by 109%, and it's projected to continue to grow annually (Kueakomoldej et al., 2021). When compared with physicians, NPs are more likely to work in rural or underserved areas, whereas the number of physicians practicing in rural and low-income areas has decreased. Even with an increase in the numbers of NPs practicing in these areas, there continues to be a shortage of healthcare providers. This scarcity has been attributed to difficulty recruiting and retaining providers, including NPs, in rural areas. Factors associated with the recruitment and retention of NPs to rural or underserved areas include individual NPs' background, NP education programs offering underserved experience and loan repayment, organizations employing NPs, the communities the NPs practice, and the ability to practice at their full scope (Kueakomoldej et al., 2021).

Rural Americans have poorer health outcomes than their urban counterparts. As a result, CMS framed several initiatives that included remote evaluation of recorded images sent by patients to their provider, expansion of Medicare to include telehealth and other virtual services, expanding the scope of practice for nonphysician providers for primary care in hospitals, and increasing the wage index of rural hospitals to enhance recruitment (Johnston et al., 2019). Many small communities struggled to recruit physicians, especially during a global health crisis. Housing shortages and government and business shutdowns made relocation difficult, if not impossible, for many, including healthcare providers. Even if providers were interested in rural practice, there were some communities that struggled with housing. Communities in the Northwest have had providers interested in taking positions at their rural hospitals. Although they were ready to sign a contract, when they met with a realtor, they found that they couldn't buy a house due to limited housing availability. The professionals who interviewed wanted to accept the job; however, because there was no housing available, this led to them to decline the position. Housing continues to be a problem due to limited infrastructure, building costs, and material availability.

This contributes to the increasing disparity of rural residents' health status. Johnston et al. (2019) found that rural residents with chronic conditions had higher preventable hospitalization and mortality rates. The pandemic also decreased access to specialists for rural residents. A rise in the supply of medical specialists lowered the mortality rate by 8.3%, and if the patient had an opportunity for one or more visits with a specialist in addition to one or more visits with a primary care provider (PCP), this reduced the preventable hospitalization rate by 15.9% and the mortality rate by 16.6% (Johnston et al., 2019).

One modest proposal to increase the number of specialist and PCPs is by using APRNs. APRNs are certified in various areas, including primary and acute care and psychiatric mental health. Buerhaus (2019) reports that patients who obtained their primary care from NPs received higher-quality care than those treated by physicians in several scenarios. Utilizing APRNs to deliver primary care will help with the physician deficiency in health professional shortage areas (HPSAs). HPSAs are generally defined as areas with a population-to-physician ratio of 3,500 to one (Marsh et al., 2012). With many graduating physicians choosing specialty areas other than family practice or primary care, the pool for potential medical doctors (MDs) to settle in rural and remote settings lessens even more. With the greater number of APRNs, especially NPs who assume a PCP role, there is the potential to improve health outcomes and reduce costs in several ways for rural and remote populations.

The emergence of APRNs started in 1965. By 2008, 8.3% of registered nurses were prepared as APRNs in one or more specialties (Marsh et al., 2012) with the number increasing. In 2009, approximately 18% of APRNs practiced in rural or frontier areas; this number is also increasing. APRNs are a good choice for offering health care to rural Americans. However, there are challenges to APRNs' rural practice, including the issue of their reimbursement, as when APRNs bill independently, they are reimbursed at a rate that is 85% of the physician reimbursement rate. However, when APRNs' services are billed under physicians, the rate is 100%, creating an incentive for "incident-to" services (Marsh et al., 2012). The hospital benefits as it is receiving full Medicare payment while paying the APRN a significantly lower salary than that of an MD. This creates an incentive for the hospital to employ APRNs. Multiple studies over the past 40 years have found that APRNs' patient outcomes are as good as those of physicians, and they often have higher patient satisfaction scores (Marsh et al., 2012). Rural access to care can be expanded by using APRNs in primary, acute, and transitional care.

The use of APRNs as PCPs was supported by the ACA, which established a grant program to fund the cost of nurse-managed health clinics. For clinics to receive funding, they needed to use APRNs as PCPs, providing care and wellness services without regard for patients' ability to pay for the services, and the clinics needed to create a community advisory committee (Marsh et al., 2012).

The pandemic has had an impact on rural health care providers. Prior to the pandemic, rural providers were overextended and experienced burnout. Caregiver fatigue continued throughout the pandemic, largely due to a shortage of providers and an aging population, factors that were significantly affected by COVID-19. Rural providers experienced burnout at a fast rate then their urban counterparts. (Terry et al., 2021). In a study that looked at the impact of the pandemic on rural healthcare providers, Terry et al. (2021) found that the greatest effect was in the areas of psychological well-being and professional and financial worries; however, job satisfaction and perceived stress were not significantly different from how they were viewed before the pandemic. Considering the associations among leadership, caregivers, and the healthcare team, the pandemic required healthcare leaders to communicate more purposefully with staff and offer mental health support (Terry et al., 2021). The study noted that improved communication and services improved the healthcare teams' culture and caregiver-leadership relations; they identified more positive than negative impacts on rural caregivers due to the pandemic (Terry et al., 2021).

Conclusion

Over the past decade, there has been an increase in the number of rural hospital closures. The impact of the COVID-19 pandemic is expected to lead to an increase in rural hospital closures and a decrease in the number of rural healthcare providers. Rural hospitals received federal funding during the pandemic, but the question remains, was the funding enough to assist rural hospitals in providing care to their communities? However, with the shift in rural health care due to the addition of increases in federal funding; the emergence of APRNs who are willing to care for rural populations; and telehealth services such as E-Hospitalist, which allows APRNs to provide care while actively consulting with a physician at a different location, these closures could possibly be reduced.

Case Study 4.1

1. How did COVID-19 change patient acuity in rural healthcare settings? Has the number of deaths increased in these settings because of the spread of COVID-19 throughout rural areas? Are these settings better equipped with personnel and equipment to care for these high acuity patients?
2. Are rural settings better equipped to care for patients with behavioral health needs? Should funding be made available for pilot studies regarding the most effective and efficient methods to provide care for individuals struggling with these needs?
3. Should funding be made available in rural areas for pilot studies regarding the most effective and efficient methods to provide care for individuals struggling with the long-term physical and emotional complications associated with COVID-19?

Case Study 4.2

1. Describe the potential opportunities and challenges for nursing and healthcare staff who are working within a setting that utilizes E-Hospitalist's services.
2. Discuss how the public's trust may be affected in settings that utilize an E-Hospitalist model of care delivery.

References

Administration for Strategic Preparedness & Response. (n.d.). *Declarations of a public health emergency*. https://aspr.hhs.gov/legal/PHE/Pages/default.aspx

American Hospital Association. (2023). *CMS issues hospital IPPS final rule for FY 2024*. https://www.aha.org/news/headline/2023-08-01-cms-issues-hospital-ipps-final-rule-fy-2024#:~:text=The%20Centers%20for%20Medicare%20%26%20Medicaid,and%20submit%20quality%20measure%20data.

Buerhaus, P. (2019). Nurse practitioners: A solution to America's primary care crisis. *Missouri State Board of Nursing, 21*(1), 16–23.

Center for Healthcare Quality and Payment Reform. (2023). *Rural hospitals at risk of closing*.

Centers for Medicare & Medicaid Services. (2023). *Medicare Program: Hospital Outpatient Prospective Payment and Ambulatory Surgical Center Payment Systems; Quality Reporting Programs; Payment for Intensive Outpatient Services in Hospital Outpatient Departments, Community Mental Health Centers, Rural Health Clinics, Federally Qualified Health Centers, and Opioid Treatment Programs; Hospital Price Transparency; Changes to Community Mental Health Centers Conditions of Participation, Changes to the Inpatient Prospective Payment System Medicare Code Editor; Rural Emergency Hospital Conditions of Participation Technical Correction*. https://federalregister.gov/d/2023-24293

Dreher, A. (2022). *Rural hospitals again face financial jeopardy*. Axios. https://www.axios.com/2022/07/14/rural-hospitals-face-financial-jeopardy

Ellison, A. (2022). *State-by-state breakdown of 76 hospital closures*. Becker's Hospital Review. https://www.beckershospitalreview.com/finance/state-by-state-breakdown-of-76-hospital-closures.html

Frieden, J. (2022, June 29). *What will ensure rural hospitals' survival? More $$ and good broadband, experts say*. Medpage Today. https://www.medpagetoday.com/practicemanagement/reimbursement/99515

Germack, H. D., Kandrack, R., & Martsolf, G. R. (2019). When rural hospitals close, the physician workforce goes away. *Health Affairs, 38*(12), 2086–2094. https://doi.org/10.1377/hlthaff.2019.00918

Johnston, K. J., Wen, H., & Joynt Maddox, K. E. (2019). Lack of access to specialists associated with mortality and preventable hospitalizations of rural Medicare beneficiaries. *Health Affairs, 38*(12), 1993–2002. https://doi.org/10.1377/hlthaff.2019.00838

Kanter, G. P., Segal, A. G., & Groeneveld, P. W. (2020). Income disparities in access to critical care services. *Health Affairs, 39*(8), 1362–1367.

Khullar, D., Bond, A. M., & Schpero, W. L. (2020). COVID-19 and the financial health of US hospitals. *Journal of American Medical Association, 323*(21), 2127–2028.

Kueakomoldej, S., Turi, E., McMenamin, A., Xue, Y., & Poghosyan, L. (2022). Recruitment and retention of primary care nurse practitioners in underserved areas: A scoping review. *Nursing Outlook, 70*(3), 401–416. https://doi.org/10.1016/j.outlook.2021.12.008

Marsh, L., Diers, D., & Jenkins, A. (2012). A modest proposal. *Policy, Politics, & Nursing Practice, 13*(4), 184–194. https://doi.org/10.1177/1527154412472710

Mosley, D., DeBehnke, D., Gaskell, S., & Weil, A. (2020, April). *Trends in rural hospital financial viability, community essentiality, and patient outmigration.* Guidehouse. https://guidehouse.com/-/media/www/site/insights/healthcare/2020/guidehouse-navigant-2020-rural-analysis.pdf

Robertson, M. (2023, January 6). *100 hospitals with the worst margins nationwide, ranked.* Becker's Hospital CEO Report. https://www.beckershospitalreview.com/finance/101-hospitals-with-the-worst-margins-nationwide-ranked.html

Rodriquez, R. M. (2020). Tackling another COVID-19 pandemic disparity: Distance from major academic medical centers encumbers emergency and critical care physician surge capacity. *Academic Emergency Medicine, 27*(11), 1212–1214.

Suttle, A. (2019). *Rural America faces a healthcare access crisis.* Modern Healthcare. https://www.modernhealthcare.com/opinion-editorial/rural-america-faces-a-healthcare-access-crisis

Terry, D. L., Hui, P., & Buntoro, S. (2021). The initial positive and negative impacts of the COVID-19 pandemic on rural healthcare providers: Associations with team culture and leadership. *Journal of Healthcare Management, 66*(5), 396–406. https://doi.org/10.1097/jhm-d-20-00258

University of North Carolina at Chapel Hill, Cecil G. Sheps Center for Health Services Research. (n.d.). *Rural hospital closures.* https://www.shepscenter.unc.edu/programs-projects/rural-health/rural-hospital-closures/

U.S. Government Accountability Office. (2018). *Rural hospital closures: Number and characteristics of affected hospitals and contributing factors.* https://www.gao.gov/products/gao-18-634.

Wishner, J., Solleveld, P., Rudowitz, R., Paradise, J., & Antonisse, L. (2016). *A look at rural hospital closures and implications for access to care: Three case studies.* Kaiser Family Foundation. https://files.kff.org/attachment/issue-brief-a-look-at-rural-hospital-closures-and-implications-for-access-to-care

UNIT III

Ambulatory Services

The COVID-19 pandemic heightened the need to address access to health care in the United States, including rural America. Many healthcare providers left their professions during this time, either taking an early retirement, making a career change, or simply quitting to avoid uncertain and unpleasant times. This exodus drove the shortage in services provided by providers in public health, mental wellness, and occupational health and rehabilitation. This was even more acute in rural and remote areas in the United States.

CHAPTER 5

Public Health Nursing's Role

The core of all public health departments is the public health nurse. For decades there has been a limited number of public health nurses (PHNs) caring for the residents in rural America (Figure 5.1). In a study conducted in 2002, it was noted that Montana, Wyoming, and Alaska together have 99 local health departments caring for almost 2,000,000 residents in rural areas; there was one full-time equivalent public health nurse for every 6,000 residents (Rosenblatt et al., 2002). Over the past 3 decades, PHN positions have been underfunded, left vacant, eliminated, or replaced. Since 2008, national, state, and local health departments have lost 55,000 public health workers, or 25% of the workforce, with PHNs being the largest segment of the group (Edmonds et al., 2020). The impact of the pandemic was exacerbated in rural communities due to contributing factors such as a declining rural population, economic stagnation, provider shortages, and older and poor residents who are underinsured and have higher rates of chronic illnesses (Melvin et al., 2020).

PHNs had a large impact on the response to the COVID-19 pandemic by serving on mobile strike teams, investigating case contacts, and delivering education based on the rapidly shifting guidance from the Centers for Disease Control and Prevention (CDC). The COVID-19 pandemic has brought public health and the need for PHNs to the forefront. The role of public health and PHNs ensures the delivery of equitable health care in rural communities. The Association of Public Health Nurses (APHN, 2022) defines *public health nursing* as "the practice of promoting and protecting the health of populations using knowledge from nursing, social, and public health sciences. Public health nursing practice focuses on population health, with the goal of promoting health, and preventing disease and disability" (p. 1). PHNs work in a variety of settings:

- schools
- health departments
- home health settings
- community health centers
- correctional facilities
- worksites, even out of mobile vans

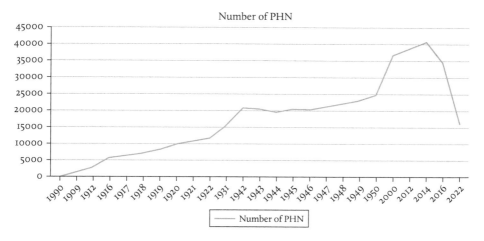

Number of PHN

FIGURE 5.1   Number of public health nurses in the United States.

School Nurse

The American Academy of Pediatrics (Korioth, 2020) has been concerned about the adverse health consequences of school closures due to COVID-19. Some of the health consequences that led to the recommendation to continue with in-person classes for students were abuse, depression, monitoring and addressing food insecurities (Abdurahman et al., 2019), and suicidal ideation. However, continuing with in-person classes and returning to school came with risks such as exposing faculty, staff, and family members to COVID-19. In a study conducted by Hoke et al. (2021) on understanding the impacts of the COVID-19 pandemic on school nurses' perceived risk, concern for returning to school, role in communities, and changes to nursing, a sample of 350 school nurses throughout Pennsylvania completed a self-reported survey, including questions evaluating their perspectives about the impact of the COVID-19 pandemic on their personal and professional practices and involvement in their school community. Specifically, they were interested in understanding how the COVID-19 pandemic was perceived and how the pandemic impacted rural versus urban schools. They determined urban school nurses were more concerned about returning to the school building without a COVID-19 vaccine than rural nurses as they were extremely concerned about their safety. It was also noted that urban nurses were more willing to get a COVID-19 vaccine when available.

The effects of the pandemic have undoubtedly highlighted the unique position of school nurses. The National Association of School Nurses (Maughan et al., 2016, p. 48) states the role of the school nurse is to advocate for policy, system, and environmental change to facilitate a healthier community. The pandemic has highlighted the need for schools, school nurses, and stakeholders on the importance of education and community engagement to improve social distancing practices during pandemics. As a result of the pandemic, the role of the school nurse has evolved, requiring them to have the ability to rapidly adjust to changing environments and be more aware of the connection a school nurse has between health care and the school community—a critical link in supporting community public health. "School nurses need to be involved in school disaster preparedness planning and activities since they are the ones who are responsible for implementing policies and programs to prevent infection transmission in schools" (Hoke et al., 2021, p. 294).

The voice of the school nurse is important in planning for ongoing school health and safety protocols. Due to the pandemic and the position school nurses fill, school communities may now be ready to listen more than ever to make evidence-based decisions to protect student and school employee safety. To be able to assume these new responsibilities, understanding that there is a shortage of these professionals as well as that their needed support and resources are imperative for success must be realized.

School nurses play a critical role in the health and wellness of school-aged children when there is not the opportunity for traditional health care. It is well known that school nurses have been overburdened and under-resourced for decades. Even before the COVID-19 pandemic, school nurses faced challenges, including inadequate time to complete all job tasks; limited resources to address student needs, especially students with chronic illness; high workload related to being responsible for students at multiple locations; and pressure from school administration. These challenges increased during the pandemic, raising concerns about school nurses' physical and mental well-being.

Fortunately, the pandemic has shed some light on the needs and requirements of school nurses through research and news articles. An analysis of articles published from February 2020 to September 2021 was conducted by Lowe et al. (2022) to explore COVID-19 occupational changes and the impact of the pandemic on school nurses and unlicensed assistive personnel (UAP) in the United States. They concluded (Figure 5.2) that during the

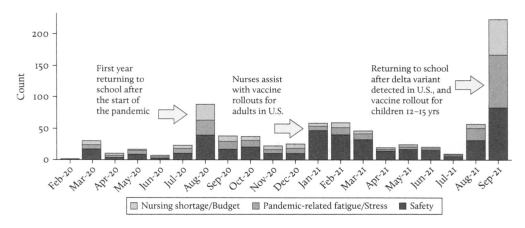

FIGURE 5.2 Themes of news articles from February 2020 to September 2021.

CASE STUDY 5.1

Gabiel is a teacher in a rural area in Virginia, where many of the students receive daily school lunches due to food insecurities. Prior to the pandemic students received breakfast and lunches, with most receiving the meals at no cost. Other students also received meals; however, due to their parents' income they were required to pay a fee, but because the financial impact of the pandemic, the cost was being covered by the school. This and the increase of the cost of food lead to a school lunch debt of more than $40,000. Knowing that the community, including the school, could not continue to cover the cost, Gabriel reached out to local nonprofit organizations and other donors and raised more than $40,000. He stated, "When I see students ... the first question I ask them isn't 'Hey are you OK? How are you?' It's 'Did you eat today?' Because a majority of the time, they're not eating" (Brumbaugh, 2023, para. 3).

pandemic, the role and responsibilities of school nurses and UAPs changed dramatically. New responsibilities included COVID-19 mitigation strategies, screening for symptoms, testing students and staff, contact tracing and data collection, and implementation of COVID-19 guidelines and protocols for their schools. The review included 496 articles; three major themes were identified:

- safety
- pandemic-related fatigue/stress
- nursing shortage/budget

The occupational challenges school nurses faced during the pandemic affected their level of stress and fatigue. This stress and fatigue ultimately affect school nurse retention and their ability to care for students in schools and communities. "School nurses play a critical role in disease surveillance, disaster preparedness, wellness and chronic disease prevention interventions, immunizations, mental health screening and chronic disease education" (Lowe et al., 2022, p. 14).

Health Department

Many PHNs work for government agencies caring for patients in state and local health departments. PHNs working at local health departments (LHDs) fulfill a variety of roles, such as conducting epidemiological research related to outbreaks, developing immunization clinics, and overseeing public health emergency preparedness programs. LHDs fulfill their role by ensuring that appropriate and effective services are available to the underserved, that policy work addresses public health issues, and that programs are implemented to promote population health. Unfortunately, decreased public health funding has prevented LHDs from carrying out their mission to promote the public's health.

The COVID-19 pandemic has had a negative impact on LHDs, which have highlighted the inequities in health and health care in the United States. In the past, research studies were conducted to explore the relationship between public health spending and health outcomes, while other studies focused on partnerships, staffing, and service. Research has determined that when an LHD is led by nurse lead executives, LHD performance increases. But what is the impact on population health? A recent study examined the relationships between the type of public health leadership and whether the lead executive was a nurse and there were changes in 15- to 44-year-olds all-cause mortality, infant mortality, and the percentage of the population with late or no entry into prenatal care (Kett et al., 2022). This research demonstrated that the presence of a nurse lead executive was associated with a 5.2% lower 15- to 44-year-old mortality rate in the Black population as well as a 6% lower Black–White mortality ratio and a reduction in the percentage of the population with late or no entry to prenatal care.

Home Health Settings

Home health nursing is rapidly growing due to the demand in services as the U.S. population ages. In 2019, there were approximately 2.3 million home care workers in the United States (Tyler et al., 2021). Home health nurses offer one-on-one care in a patient's home, allowing the patient to remain with their family in a familiar setting. The COVID-19 pandemic reshaped home care services and policies that related to the provision of home care with staffing shortages, increased risk of infection due to lack of personal protective equipment (PPE), and inadequate training, which impacted home health agencies and their staff.

Staffing in home care agencies was already problematic before the pandemic, and staffing shortages worsened during and after. Many staff left their jobs due to fear of exposure to the virus, especially in the first 3 to 6 months of the pandemic when there was difficulty accessing PPE. Some older workers and people with underlying conditions that made them more susceptible to hospitalization if exposed to COVID-19 chose to leave the field or retire. The closure of schools and childcare centers was another burden for home health care workers as they were not able to find childcare. Nurses reported tremendous new challenges and danger due to the pandemic with fear of infection, exhaustion from heavy workloads, and the stress of nursing seriously ill COVID-19 patients (Liu et al., 2020).

The COVID-19 outbreak also caused substantial changes in the competencies of home care nurses. Their workload increased considerably, so workflow and responsibilities were constantly being readjusted. Rotating shifts were implemented to carry out diagnosis and follow-up of patients infected by COVID-19 and for the care of home patients. To ensure all patients received the treatment needed, many aspects of home care were delegated to family caregivers (Ruiz-Fernandez et al., 2022), without time or resources to correctly train the family member proficiently.

Home care agencies and state and federal governments addressed some of these issues through changes to policies, regulations, and guidance. However, due to differences in the definition of essential workers, several states did not recognize home health workers as essential workers, which resulted in difficulty in obtaining PPE, testing for COVID-19, and accessing the vaccine. This contributed to many workers leaving their position for fear of contracting the virus.

Home health agencies quickly addressed challenges and took advantage of federal and state policy changes and regulations such as increased telehealth opportunities, CARES Act funding, the Paycheck Protection Program (PPP), and the Families First Coronavirus Relief Act (FFCRA) to pay workers retainers, bonuses, and hazard pay and to pay them for time spent sick or quarantining after exposure (Tyler et al., 2021). The CARES Act also provided for the use of telehealth by home health agencies. However, in March of 2020, CMS clarified the Interim Final Rule that it could not reimburse home health providers for these services due to a statutory provision that prohibited visits via telecommunications technology from being considered as equivalent to in-person visits (Tyler et al., 2021). Despite the inability to bill for telehealth visits, many agencies reported adding telehealth services to obtain signatures and consents or interview prospective employees as well as to continue to provide care and monitor clients remotely, from providing medication reminders to conducting physical therapy sessions over video applications. Agencies developed tools, such as apps, to screen their staff and their clients on a regular basis and monitor COVID-19 exposure, symptoms, or any high-risk travel. Agencies also used technology to communicate with and support family caregivers in the absence of home health workers. Most telehealth services were conducted telephonically, which did not involve adding telehealth infrastructure.

There were also changes to staff training, qualifications, and duties to increase the number of available home health workers. Thirty-two states made changes to their pre-employment requirements to increase the number of employees and to retain current employees. State policy changes were made such as hazard pay and retainer payments (Tyler et al., 2021). These payments were made for staff who were at risk of contracting COVID-19 during work or if they had to quarantine after exposure. Nineteen states utilized hazard payment or add-on payments for workers, and 27 states implemented retainer payments (Figure 5.3).

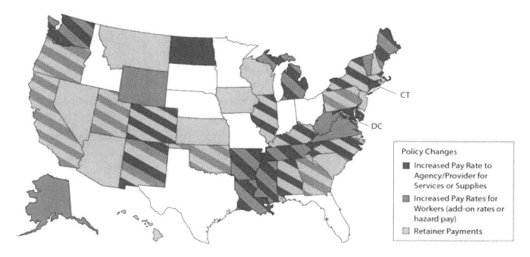

FIGURE 5.3 State policy changes related to increased Medicaid payment rates to home care agencies or workers.

In addition to the threat to physical safety, there were inconsistent training requirements that made it difficult to recruit staff from other health care sectors due to different training and certification requirements. Some states temporarily relaxed the training requirements, which led to uncertainty that the staff hired under these conditions would eventually be required to complete the appropriate training (Figure 5.4).

As a result of the number of workers who left home care positions, there was a change in client loads, which resulted in staffing challenges. At the beginning of the pandemic,

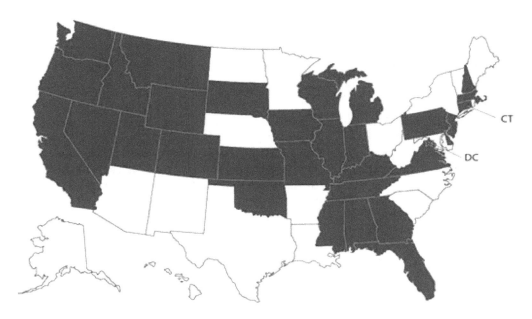

FIGURE 5.4 State policy changes related to employment requirements and qualifications for home care workers.

clients were afraid to have others outside of their immediate family in their homes for fear of exposure. Many clients who did not have life-threatening needs opted to receive care from family members (Figure 5.5), especially family members who were working from home. Some of these family members even received payment for the care they provided. According to Mauro et al. (2020), patients' fear of being infected contributed to reducing the demand for care. But the interruption in routine service care led to increased morbidity and mortality in older people with complex chronic conditions (Krist et al., 2020). The initial decline in demand for home health and home care services has returned to full client loads, with most returning to normal by the beginning of 2021 (Tyler et al., 2021).

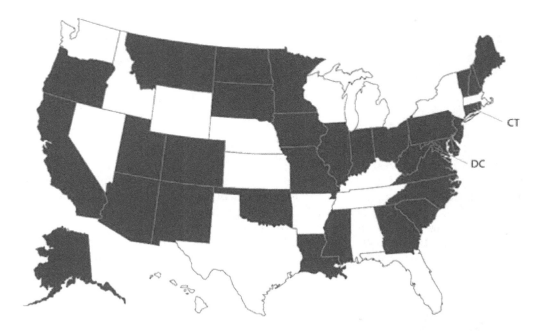

FIGURE 5.5 State policy changes allowing payment or increased payments to family caregivers.

The impact of the COVID-19 pandemic on home health care has led to recommendations for changes such as the assurance that home care workers are designated as essential workers, which will provide them with priority access to PPE, testing, and vaccines. Wage improvement and more career opportunities through better training and career ladders and other requirements across states to make access more portable are all being considered. In addition, government reimbursement for certain telehealth services is needed.

Community Health Centers

Community health centers (CHCs) in rural areas fill a vital role for residents who do not have access to health care services. In their role, CHCs treat patients with urgent illnesses, manage chronic conditions, provide immunizations, and educate patients on preventive care, health, and wellness. They may perform pregnancy testing along with pregnancy counseling or sexually transmitted infection testing and tracing.

CHCs played a key role in the national, state, and local responses to the pandemic, particularly in rural areas. In 2020, CHCs tested more than 3.7 million patients for the coronavirus and cared for nearly 745,000 patients diagnosed with COVID-19 (Sharac et al., 2022). These health centers served more than 30 million patients in 2021, the largest number of patients recorded since the first CHC was opened (Sharac et al., 2022). During the pandemic, a portion of these visits were telehealth visits. In 2021, 26 million visits to CHCs were telehealth, representing 21% of all visits (Sharac et al., 2022). This was an increase of 20% over the number of telehealth visits in 2019 (Figure 5.6). Medical, mental health, and substance used disorder (SUD) visits also increased compared to prepandemic levels (Figure 5.7). Mental health visits rose by 19% from 2019 to 2021 as a result of telehealth services (Sharac et al., 2022). However, during this time, dental and vision visits remained below prepandemic visits as these services cannot be offered via telehealth. Along with lower dental and vision visits, there also was a lower level of children seen by CHCs. From 2019 to 2021 there was a decrease of 6%, and the number of children served at school-based clinics declined by 13% (Figure 5.8).

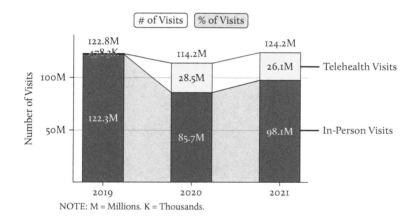

FIGURE 5.6 Telehealth and in-person visits to CHCs, 2019–2021.

CHCs experienced a demand for mental health service. From 2019 to 2021 there was an increase in mental health visits by 19% due to the increase in the number of patients experiencing anxiety disorders. The number of patients receiving medication-assisted treatment (MAT) for opioid use disorder (OUD) treatment also increased over the same period, with an increase of 29% representing 180,000 patients (Figure 5.9).

National trends indicate that there were fewer CHCs patients who were uninsured in 2021 compared to prepandemic levels. This was a drop in the number of uninsured patients at CHCs from 2019 to 2021 by 10%. This drop was due in part to temporary policies ensuring continuous Medicaid enrollment during the pandemic. As a result of continuous enrollment there was an increase in the number of Medicaid patients seen (2%), with Medicaid/Children's Health Insurance Program being the largest source of coverage, 49% of patients (Figure 5.10).

In total, CHCs received $2.8 billion in pandemic-related funding in 2021 that enabled centers to address the changing health care needs of their patients by offering telehealth and mental health services. Unfortunately, this funding has expired, resulting in increased challenges for CHCs as they continue to try and address all the varied needs for their many patients.

Medical Services

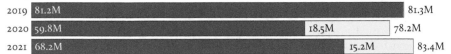

2019	81.2M	81.3M
2020	59.8M	18.5M	78.2M
2021	68.2M	15.2M	83.4M

Dental Services

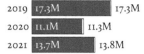

2019	17.3M	17.3M
2020	11.1M	11.3M
2021	13.7M	13.8M

Integrated Mental Health Services

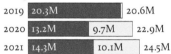

2019	20.3M	20.6M
2020	13.2M	9.7M	22.9M
2021	14.3M	10.1M	24.5M

Integrated SUD Services

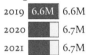

2019	6.6M	6.6M
2020		6.7M
2021		6.7M

Vision Services

2019	1.1M
2020	788.8K
2021	1M

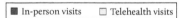

■ In-person visits   ☐ Telehealth visits

NOTE: SUD = Substance use disorder. Social supportive services (also called "enabling services") not shown. It is possible that people can receive multiple services in a single visit to a health center, and so the sum of visits across services do not sum to the total visits shown in Figure 1. Integrated Mental Health visits include some mental health services provided by medical providers and are counted in both categories. Integrated SUD visits include some SUD services provided by either mental health or medical providers and are counted in both categories.

FIGURE 5.7 Telehealth and in-person visits for selected services at CHCs, 2019–2021.

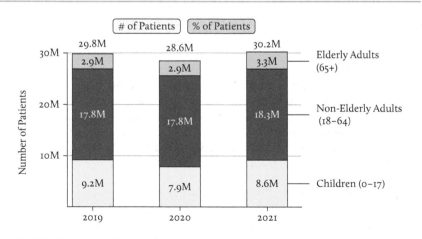

FIGURE 5.8 Health center patients by age group, 2019–2021.

Patients with Selected Mental Health Diagnoses

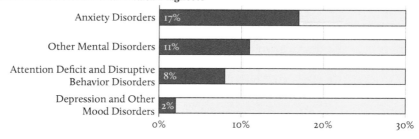

Patients with Selected SUD Diagnoses

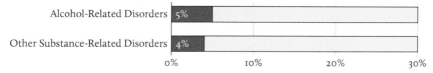

Patients Receiving Selected SUD Service

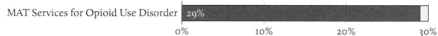

NOTE: MAT = Medication-Assisted Treatment. SUD = Substance Use Disorder. Other Substance- Related Disorder excludes alcohol-related and tobacco use disorder. In 2021, there were 3,007,893 patients diagnosed with anxiety disorders, 2,112,464 patients diagnosed with other mental disorders, 643,092 patients diagnosed with attention deficit and disruptive behavior disorders, 2,722,720 patients diagnosed with depression and other mood disorders, 402,991 patients with alcohol-related disorders, 665,130 patients with other substance-related disorders, and 184,379 patients receiving MAT for opioid use disorder.

FIGURE 5.9 Percent change in the number of health center patients with selected diagnoses or receiving MAT for OUD, 2019–2021.

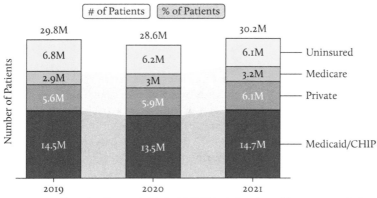

NOTE: M = Millions. K = Thousands. Medicaid/CHIP includes other public insurance, which made up less than 1% of patients.

FIGURE 5.10 Health coverage among health center patients, 2019–2021.

Conclusion

PHNs have a large impact on the response to the COVID-19 pandemic and the long-term effects of the illness. During the pandemic, PHNs served on mobile strike teams, investigated case contacts, and delivered education based on the rapidly shifting guidance from the CDC. The COVID-19 pandemic has brought public health and the need for PHNs to the forefront. The role of public health and PHNs ensures the delivery of equitable health care in rural communities. The impact of the pandemic was exacerbated in rural communities due to contributing factors such as a declining rural population, economic stagnation, provider shortages, and older and low-income residents who are underinsured and who have higher rates of chronic illnesses (Melvin et al., 2020).

The response to the COVID-19 pandemic highlights the U.S. public health system and health equity challenges as well as the importance of including nurses and a nursing perspective when addressing public health issues. However, we need to increase nurse visibility. Nurses possess a variety of transferable skills for public health development (Morone et al., 2022). "Increasing the visibility of nurses will require collective promotion of the profession as a source of credible and competent expertise in promoting the health of communities and populations across settings including the academic, community, health system, and policy arenas" (Morone et al., 2022, p. S235).

Questions for Discussion Related to Case Study 5.1

1. What other avenues could Gabriel take to cover the cost of the meals at his school?
2. Discuss how Gabriel can lobby for changes to lunch programs to address food insecurities. What approach do you recommend?
3. Define *food insecurities* and how they impact student learning and development.

References

Abdurahman, A. A., Chaka, E. E., Nedjat, S., Dorosty, A. R., & Majzadeh, R. (2019). The association of household food insecurity with the risk of type 2 diabetes mellitus in adults: A systematic review and meta-analysis. *European Journal of Nutrition, 58*(4), 1341–1350. https://doi.org/10.1007/s00394-018-1705-2

Association of Public Health Nurses. (2022). *Home page.* https://www.phnurse.org

Brumbaugh, J. (2023, April 27). Teacher raises over $40,000 to pay his school's entire student lunch debt. *Herndon Observer.* https://www.mynbc5.com/article/teacher-raises-money-to-pay-school-student-lunch-debt/43703453#

Edmonds, J. K., Kneipp, S. M., & Campbell, L. (2020). A call to action for public health nurses during the COVID-19 pandemic. *Public Health Nursing, 37*(3), 323–324. https://doi.org/10.1111/phn.12733

Hoke, A. M., Keller, C. M., Calo, W. A., Sekhar, D. L., Lehman, E. B., & Kraschnewski, J. L. (2021). School nurse perspectives on COVID-19. *The Journal of School Nursing, 37*(4), 292–297.

Kett, P., Bekemeier, B., Herting, J. & Altman, M. (2022). Addressing health disparities: The health department nurse lead executive's relationship to improved community health. *Journal of Public Health Management and Practice, 28*(2), E566–E576. https://doi.org/10.1097/PHH.0000000000001425

Korioth, T. (2020, June 26). *AAP interim guidance on school re-entry focuses on mitigating COVID-19 risks*. American Academy of Pediatrics. https://publications.aap.org/aapnews/news/6706/AAP-interim-guidance-on-school-re-entry-focuses-on?autologincheck=redirected

Krist, A. H., DeVoe, J. E., Cheng, A., Ehrlich, T., & Jones, S. M. (2020). Redesigning primary care to address the COVID-19 pandemic in the midst of the pandemic. *Annals of Family Medicine, 18*, 349–354. https://doi.org/10.1370/afm.2557

Kub, J., Kulbok, P. A., & Glick, D. (2015). Cornerstone documents, milestones, and policies: Shaping the direction of public health nursing, 1890–1950. *OJIN: The Online Journal of Issues in Nursing, 20*(2), 1890–1950.

Liu, Y.-E., Zhai, Z.-C., Han, Y.-H., Liu, Y.-L., Liu, F.-P., & Hu, D.-Y. (2020). Experiences of frontline nurses combating coronavirus disease—2019 in China: A qualitative analysis. *Public Health Nursing, 37*, 757–763. https://doi.org/10.1111/phn.12768

Lowe, A. A., Ravi, P., Gerald, L. B, & Wilson, A.M. (2022). The changing job of school nurse during the COVID-19 pandemic: A media content analysis of contribution to stress. *Annals of Work Exposures and Health, 67*(1), 1–17.

Maughan, E. D., Bobo, N., Butler, S., & Schantz, S. (2016). Framework for 21st Century School Nursing Practice: National Association of School Nurses. NASN School Nurse, 31(1), 45–53. https://doi.org/10.1177/1942602X15618644

Mauro, V., Lorenzo, M., Paolo, C., & Sergio, H. (2020). Treat all COVID-19-positive patients, but do not forget those negative with chronic diseases. *Internal and Emergency Medicine, 15*, 787–790. https://doi.org/10.1007/s11739-020-02395-z

Melvin, S. C., Wiggins, C., Burse, N., Thompson, E., & Monger, M. (2020). The role of public health in COVID-19 emergency response efforts from a rural health perspective. *Preventing Chronic Disease, 17*, 200–256.

Morone, J. F., Tolentino, D. A., Aronowitz, S. V., Siddiq, H. (2022). The COVID-19 pandemic and the push to promote and include nurses in public health policy. *American Journal of Public Health, 112*(S3), 231–236. https://doi.org/10.2105/AJPH.2022.306837

Rosenblatt, R. A., Casey, S., & Richardson, M. (2002). Rural-urban differences in the public health workforce: Local health departments in 3 rural Western states. *American Journal of Public Health, 92*(7), 1102–1105. https://www.ncbi.nlm.nih.gov/pmc/articles/PMC1447195/pdf/0921102.pdf

Ruiz-Fernandez, M. D., Fernandez-Medina, I. M., Ramirez, F. G., Granero-Molina, J., Fernandez-Sola, C., & Hernandez-Padilla, J. M. (2022). Experiences of home care nurses during the COVID-19 pandemic. *Nursing Research, 71*(2), 111–118.

Sharac, J., Corallo, B., Tolbert, J, Shin, P., & Rosenbaum, S. (2022). *Changes in community health center patients and services during the COVID-19 pandemic*. Kaiser Family Foundation. https://www.kff.org/medicaid/issue-brief/changes-in-community-health-center-patients-and-services-during-the-covid-19-pandemic/

Tyler, D., Hunter, M., Mulmule, N., & Porter, K. (June 1, 2021). *COVID-19 intensifies home care workforce challenges* [Issue brief]. Office of the Assistant Secretary for Planning and Evaluation, U.S. Department of Health and Human Services. https://aspe.hhs.gov/reports/covid-19-intensifies-home-care-workforce-challenges

Image Credits

Fig. 5.1b: Source: Angela J. Beck and Matthew L. Boulton, "The Public Health Nurse Workforce in U.S. State and Local Health Departments, 2012," Public Health Reports, vol. 131, no. 1, 2016.

Fig. 5.1c: Source: Zippia, Inc., "Public Health Nurse Demographics and Statistics in the U.S.," https://www.zippia.com/public-health-nurse-jobs/demographics/, 2023.

Fig. 5.2: Ashley A. Lowe, Priyanka Ravi, Lynn B. Gerald, and Amanda M. Wilson, "The Changing Job of School Nurses during the COVID-19 Pandemic: A Media Content Analysis of Contributions to Stress," Annals of Work Exposures and Health, vol. 67, no. 1, p. 6. Copyright © 2023 by Oxford University Press.

Fig. 5.3: Denise Tyler, Melissa Hunter, Natalie Mulmule, and Kristie Porter, "State Policy Changes Related to Increase Medicaid Payment Rates to Home Care Agencies or Workers," https://aspe.hhs.gov/reports/covid-19-intensifies-home-care-workforce-challenges#figure1, 2021.

Fig. 5.4: Denise Tyler, Melissa Hunter, Natalie Mulmule, and Kristie Porter, "State Policy Changes Related to Employment Requirements and Qualifications for Home Care Workers," https://aspe.hhs.gov/reports/covid-19-intensifies-home-care-workforce-challenges#figure2, 2021.

Fig. 5.5: Denise Tyler, Melissa Hunter, Natalie Mulmule, and Kristie Porter, "State Policy Changes Allowing Payment (or Increased Payments) to Family Caregivers," https://aspe.hhs.gov/reports/covid-19-intensifies-home-care-workforce-challenges#figure3, 2021.

Fig. 5.6: Source: https://www.kff.org/medicaid/issue-brief/changes-in-community-health-center-patients-and-services-during-the-covid-19-pandemic/.

Fig. 5.7: Source: https://www.kff.org/medicaid/issue-brief/changes-in-community-health-center-patients-and-services-during-the-covid-19-pandemic/.

Fig. 5.8: Source: https://www.kff.org/medicaid/issue-brief/changes-in-community-health-center-patients-and-services-during-the-covid-19-pandemic/.

Fig. 5.9: Source: https://www.kff.org/medicaid/issue-brief/changes-in-community-health-center-patients-and-services-during-the-covid-19-pandemic/.

Fig. 5.10: Source: https://www.kff.org/medicaid/issue-brief/changes-in-community-health-center-patients-and-services-during-the-covid-19-pandemic/.

CHAPTER 6

Vulnerable Populations and Community-Focused Care

The Occupational Safety and Health Administration (OSHA, 2021) categorizes occupational hazards as chemical, physical, and biological. This definition fails to identify psychosocial hazards and their impact on the health care workforce. However, the International Labour Organization's (2022) definition focuses on the intersection between circumstances within an organization and the worker's needs and skill abilities. The COVID-19 pandemic required that occupational health nurses address the chemical, physical, biological, and psychosocial consequences that this virus has had on health care workers, their work settings, and the affective disruptions that have the potential to cause harm for years to come (World Health Organization, 2022).

Role diffusion is necessary for rural nurses caring for patients in various settings. Rural occupational nurses must possess the didactic knowledge, skills, and attitudes required to provide care for a range of persons across multigenerations experiencing the physical, behavioral, and spiritual consequences of contracting COVID-19. Nurses working in rural settings must be competent in dealing with the complexities often associated with role diffusion. The specific roles and responsibilities they assume are influenced by the settings in which they provide care and their ability to gain acceptance from a patient population that may be spread over countless miles of challenging terrain, cultural differences, and minimal access to medical care.

Agriculture

The agricultural industry is unique in its ability to include persons of varying ages and cultures. A family-operated farm is typically organized similarly to other industries, except the workers are of different ages (Bushy, 2000). In addition to workers being of different ages, they can also be from different cultures. Many farms in the United States depend on migrant workers who travel during the year to various areas, depending on the season and crops. There are an estimated 2.9 million agricultural workers in the United States, with 70% foreign born (National Center for Farmworker Health, 2022). Migrant farm workers follow migratory patterns in the United States with three hubs in the southern United States: California, Texas, and Florida (Figure 6.1).

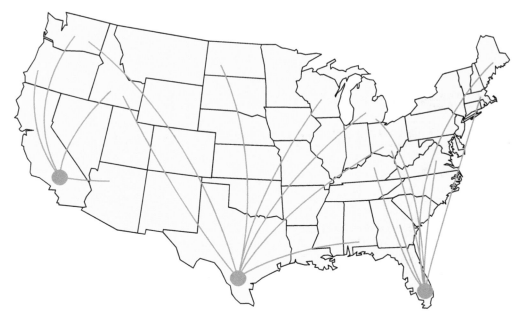

FIGURE 6.1 Migratory patterns of the United States.

Migrant farmworkers and their families have multiple challenges to accessing health care. Over two thirds of migrant households live below the poverty line while working undesirable and unsafe jobs. Their children do not have the opportunity for consistent education as migrant families move from one area to another for work, resulting in inconsistent attendance. Additionally, many children are needed to work in the fields and orchards to add to income for the family. Traveling from one area to another also impacts health. It is hard to comply with treatment for a chronic illness if you do not have consistent access to health care. Migrant workers are also subjected to overcrowded housing, unclean water, and unsanitary conditions.

During the pandemic, farm workers were established as essential as they were a key component of America's food chain. Initially spared from COVID, once the virus reached farmworkers, it spread rapidly through the migrant community as workers traveled together on crowded buses to the fields and could not afford to take time off and lose their wages (Table 6.1). For example, the number of cases tripled in just 2 weeks in Immokalee, Florida. Due to the increase in cases, the Coalition of Immokalee Workers, a nonprofit organization, advocated for local farm workers. In response, the state set up handwashing stations in the town; however, this was not enough as many federal and state recommendations were not feasible for migrant workers. Farm workers diagnosed with COVID were encouraged to isolate, which is difficult in a community where many live in crowded housing with other migrant workers. Florida provided free noncommunal housing, but it was located 40 miles away. To address the problem, Doctors Without Borders traveled to the area at the request of the Coalition of Immokalee Workers and offering testing near the farm workers' homes, as well as education and treatment in their native language. Also at the request of Doctors Without Borders, the state of Florida started to offer regular testing for anyone who wanted it, symptoms or no symptoms. It was estimated that during this time only 10% of workers were tested, with many leaving the area to work in other parts of the United States, without knowledge of their health status (Gomez, 2020, 2021).

During the height of the COVID-19 pandemic, agricultural workers organized and advocated for people experiencing symptoms of the virus to be tested and, if positive, granted paid sick leave. According to the U.S. Department of Homeland Security, these workers were considered vital to the sustainability of the food and agriculture sphere (Cybersecurity and Infrastructure Security Agency, U.S. Department of Homeland Security, 2020). However, while many other types of workers could work remotely during the initial surges of the COVID-19 pandemic, agricultural workers and rural occupational health nurses who cared for them were deemed essential despite the risks to their health and safety. Few protections were implemented by agricultural corporations, despite the government offering protection (Ávila, 2021).

TABLE 6.1 Estimated Number of Cumulative Cases and Deaths From COVID-19 Among Types of Agricultural Workers Up to March 31, 2021

Type	Cases	Case Incidence Rate	Deaths	Death Incidence Rate
Producers	329,031	9.55%	6,166	0.179%
Hired workers	170,137	9.31%	2,969	0.160%
Unpaid workers	202,902	9.39%	3,812	0.176%
Migrant workers	27,223	9.01%	459	0.152%

Source: Lusk and Chandra (2021).

The Relationship Among Nursing, Farming, and Illness

An acute, chronic, or disabling illness experienced by one member of a farming family often impacts the entire family unit, and individual family members must adapt to meet the greater needs of the family and farming responsibilities. According to Bushy (2000), both the patient and the family members who experience the consequences of a disability go through a grieving process. There is an initial denial, then anger and anxiety about the events and circumstances. There is no standard timeline for adjustment to these losses, and some family members may linger in one stage for extended time periods.

In 2003, AgriSafe (2022) was founded by rural nurses who believed that working collaboratively could improve the health and safety of farmers and ranchers. Currently, AgriSafe builds the competency of health and safety professionals to deliver best practices in agricultural health. The organization provides a vaccine confidence toolkit designed by rural nurses for rural organizations, community groups, educators, and health care providers in clinics and schools. The resource offers several downloaded graphics and templates for social media posts that are free and available to anyone interested in protecting their farming community (Figure 6.2).

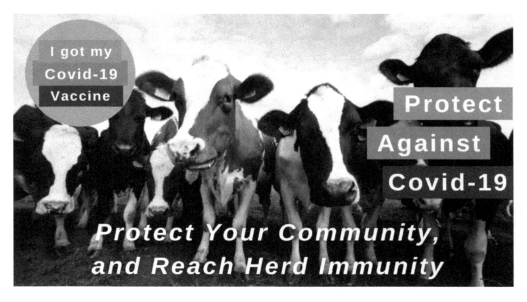

FIGURE 6.2 COVID-19 vaccination campaign poster focused on rural communities.

Javier is married and has four children. He is a migrant worker traveling with his family throughout the year depending on when crops are ready for picking. He and his family travel among Texas, Idaho, and Washington states. He considers himself lucky because when he is in all these states for work, there is housing available for not only him but his family; however, the housing is crowded. Since he travels to the same areas each year, he and his family are familiar with the areas, and they have made friends whom they can rely on if needed.

Javier was diagnosed with diabetes a few years ago. He tries his best to manage his illness, but he finds this difficult due to limited access to health care and finances. He does have a primary care provider in Texas, but he only spends 3 to 4 months in the area, so he is unable to receive treatment throughout the entire year. He tries to take the medication prescribed to him when he can afford it and will test his blood sugar only once a month because of the cost of supplies. He is concerned about his condition as he has noticed that he has developed pain in his feet and hands, which makes it hard to work, but he cannot take time off from work because he needs to support his family.

The Impact of the COVID-19 Pandemic on Persons Living With Chronic and Rare Diseases

The prolonged postponement of appointments, long waitlists, and concerns about getting infected are some unintended consequences of the COVID-19 pandemic. These challenges made it harder for people with chronic and rare illnesses in rural and remote areas to know when to seek medical care (AgriSafe, 2022).

Primary and Preventive Health Care

"Compared to urban residents, rural residents have limited access to primary healthcare, are of advanced age, and have multiple chronic conditions that have been associated with adverse COVID-19 outcomes" (Peters, 2020, p. 447). The numerous chronic illnesses that rural residents experience and rural nurses must support, combined with the higher percentage of elders, indicates the vulnerability of rural residents to acute and long-term complications from the COVID-19 virus.

A total of 14 states (primarily in the South and the Plains) have not accepted the Affordable Care Act Medicaid expansion, resulting in millions of the poorest and sickest Americans without access to health care. This contributes to many regional and local hospital closing or being at risk of closing because of the exorbitant cost of care and the high percentage of rural uninsured and underinsured people. People with COVID-19 in those states had limited access to testing and the kind of emergency and intensive care they needed (Van Dorn et al., 2020).

Pharmacologic and Nonpharmacologic Treatments

In the first few months of the COVID-19 pandemic, trends of stockpiling medications were seen. This trend, along with supply chain issues and manufacturer struggles, resulted in an 8% increase in active drug shortages in the United States in early 2020 (Clement et al., 2021). Rural residents living with multiple comorbid illnesses are particularly vulnerable to interruptions in medications when there are shortages, which were compounded by supply chain issues. But while there was an initial increase in prescription drug claims at the pandemic onset, there was a decrease in subsequent months. Clement et al. (2021) speculate that this was the result of social distancing and isolation at home. The researchers also found that there was a decline in the number of new patients starting new medication therapies from many drug classes. For the most part, many patients were able to fill medications needed for chronic health issues at the start, but as the pandemic wore on, it became a challenge. Supply chain demands and delays impacted the production and distribution of many medications and over-the-counter drugs. This resulted in many patients going without their needed prescriptions.

People living in rural settings have fewer pharmacy options. "Pharmacy deserts lead to issues of reduced access for populations in lower socioeconomic and rural locations" (Constantin et al., 2022, p. 4). If they need medications for chronic health issues, they have the option to use mail order services, but broadband access and reliability can serve as a barrier to ordering their prescriptions. Mail order services are efficient for prescriptions treating chronic conditions. However, mail order services do not provide education, screening, and other advantageous services provided by real-life pharmacists. This also is not an option for urgent medications that need to be filled and dispensed promptly and conveniently, nor for medications that are not necessarily kept in stock by mail-order firms (Constantin et al., 2022). Many must find reliable transportation if a new prescription needs to be filled for an acute incident. Because of the higher numbers of uninsured rural residents, this service might not be an option.

Telepharmacy is a possible solution to pharmacy deserts, with a pharmacist available to instruct the patient on medication actions, potential negative interactions, and side effects. A pharmacist can also oversee a pharmacy technician in communities that do not have a pharmacist. This solution could address the need to travel many miles for pharmacologics.

Testing and Medical Services Instead of Help for COVID-19

"Rural areas generally have more limited access to health care, fewer facilities, and many are on the brink of an insufficient health care infrastructure (Fahs, 2020, p. 2). Although most people infected with COVID-19 only experienced mild symptoms, some in the rare disease community said the virus made some symptoms of their rare disease worse. The expansion of telehealth services has become more available during the pandemic, which has resulted in easier-to-get care, provided residents have internet connectivity (see Chapter 7 for more information on telehealth).

Working With Victims of Human Trafficking

Individuals who experience human trafficking (U.S. Department of Homeland Security, n. d.) are also a vulnerable population. "Human trafficking is a human rights, public health, criminal justice, and health care issue" (Clemmons-Brown, 2020, p. 581). Victims of trafficking may be traced to rural and remote areas as migrant workers. Human trafficking became illegal in the United States in 2000 when the Trafficking Victims Protection Act was passed and became a federal law. During the COVID-19 pandemic, this population, like many, was overlooked due to government restrictions and shutdowns. "In 2021, the US National Human Trafficking Hotline received 50,123 signals from the Hotline. These signals include calls, texts, and online chats and tips" (National Human Trafficking Hotline, 2024, Human Trafficking Hotline Statistics section). This was a decrease compared to 2020 (56,127 signals) and 2019 (51,921 signals; National Human Trafficking Hotline, 2024).

Rural occupational health nurses have a unique opportunity to influence care for these victims if they establish a trusting relationship in the workplace. However, the spread of the COVID-19 virus has posed additional barriers to delivering trauma-informed care for this vulnerable population. These individuals were further isolated and marginalized because of governmental restrictions during the height of the closure of rural businesses and farming activities. Caring for this population requires knowledge of legal requirements for reporting and other resources (Table 6.2).

TABLE 6.2 Human Trafficking Resources

Organizations	Website
Antislavery International	antislavery.org
Coalition Against Trafficking in Women	https://catwinternational.org/
International Labour Organization	https://www.ilo.org/global/lang--en/index.htm
National Center for Missing & Exploited Children	https://www.missingkids.org/HOME
Polaris Project	https://www.polarisproject.org
Shared Hope International	https://www.sharedhope.org
U.S. Department of Health & Human Services	https://www.hhs.gov
U.S. Department of State	https://www.state.gov
United Nations Office on Drugs and Crime	https://www.unodc.org

Source: Raker (2020).

The Impact of COVID-19 on U.S. Coal Miners

Coal mines were designated as essential businesses in most states during the pandemic. The Mine Safety and Health Administration (MSHA) established regulations to decrease the spread of COVID in mines. Their recommendations included washing hands frequently, disinfecting equipment, and maintaining six feet of distance between workers. However, their recommendations were not feasible for coal miners. Coal miners work in closely packed areas. They change their clothing in packed changing rooms and ride in rail cars side by side with their coworkers, sometimes for more than an hour (Boles, 2020). Once miners reach their destinations underground, there is limited ventilation. All these occupational factors lead to an increased risk of the spread of COVID.

The first reported cases of COVID were two miners in a coal mine in Pennsylvania. Due to the inability to contact the hundreds of workers and their family members, the mine opted to close the mine for 2 weeks (Boles, 2020). Cases continued to be identified in mines throughout the United States over March and April of 2020 (Table 6.3). In April 2020, reporters were told that the MSHA was keeping a spreadsheet of COVID-related closures; however, no data has been made available to date (Tate, 2020).

TABLE 6.3 Initial Reported Cases of COVID-19 in U.S. Coal Mines

Date	Mine	Action
March 30, 2020	CONSOL Energy Inc.'s Bailey Mine, Pennsylvania	Mine shutdown for 2 weeks
	Buchanan Mine No. 1, Virginia	Mine shutdown to stop spread
	Osaka, Virginia	Mine shutdown to stop spread
	Pigeon Creek, Virginia	Mine shutdown to stop spread
	North Fork, Virginia	Mine shutdown to stop spread
April 2020	Arch Coal Inc.'s West Elk, Colorado	Mine shutdown to stop spread
	Peabody Energy's Shoal Creek, Alabama	Mine shutdown to stop spread
	Peabody Energy's Warrior Met Coal's No. 7 Mine	Mine shutdown to stop spread

Source: Tate (2020).

Contact tracing and testing for COVID-19 in mining communities is important. Coal miners are especially vulnerable to coronavirus due to lung impairment. A high percentage of miners have lung damage due to toxic coal and rock dust (Boles, 2020). While there has been a decrease in the number of cases of black lung, the number of cases have increased to epidemic levels. The National Institute for Occupational Safety and Health Epidemiologists estimates that one in five experienced coal miners in Appalachia have some degree of black lung. In the United States, according to the CDC, about 10% of coal miners have been diagnosed with black lung disease (Wade, 2020). The USA Coal Miners Union stated in March of 2020 that "black-lung coal miners *are* facing a serious threat from virus spread" (Wade, 2020, para. 1, emphasis in original). The coal mining industry was in sharp decline when the pandemic hit, which led to mass layoffs; the impact of the coronavirus has increased the number of mines that have closed either temporarily or for good.

Strategies for Addressing Vaccine Hesitancy

The Colorado Community Engagement Alliance Against COVID-19 Disparities (CO-CEAL) research team worked with five racial/ethnic communities in Colorado to examine the reasons for COVID-19 vaccine hesitancy. The team developed community-based education that could be distributed to local residents to increase the vaccination rate. The team led by Nease et al. (2022) received funding for 1 year as a part of the national Community Engagement Alliance League (CEAL) team's effort. The researchers determined that the rapid timeline and funding stream would require adaptations to their typical approach when collaborating with community and academic settings. However, the researchers were able to effectively utilize long-term relationships that existed among this diverse community population, and they quickly established trust with the local residents. The community connectors led the recruitment efforts of local residents for community survey data collection (goal of 200 surveys from each community) and participation in five community (boot camp) Translations. The community connectors continue to disseminate information regarding COVID-19 to local residents within these diverse groups of citizens. Success of this strategy can be attributed to the depth of prior investments in building and maintaining relationships, which made a difference in how rapidly and successfully partners worked together to address a crisis like the COVID-19 pandemic (Nease et al., 2022).

Living With Multiple Comorbidities

The long-term consequences of repeated exposure to chemical emissions from industrial processing plants is a risk industrial workers and coal miners have lived with for generations. The existence of known carcinogens, such as crystalline silica, exposure to wildfire smoke, coal, welding fumes, and the COVID-19 virus, poses acute and long-term health concerns such as asthma, COPD, lung cancer, and multisystem complications of COVID-19, which can pose life-threatening challenges for occupational health nurses who must design care for these workers and their families (Birrell, 2022).

The occupational health nurse should lead initiatives that involve selecting and properly using PPE, which can significantly reduce exposure to the COVID-19 virus and occupational hazards when selected and used appropriately. In selecting PPE, the nurse must consider environmental factors, including the type of airborne contaminant, tasks, other personal equipment, and location (clinical setting, intrinsically safe areas, tight spaces, working from height; Birrell, 2022). The nurse's role includes providing care, educating, and advocating for the selection of PPE along with guidelines, standards, and regulations that advise the type, fit, and level of protection offered.

Occupational Health Nursing Care Following the Withdrawal of the COVID-19 Mandate

On January 25, 2022, the Occupational Safety & Health Administration (OSHA) withdrew the Emergency Temporary Standard (ETS) requiring vaccines and testing for private employers. Although OSHA retracted the ETS, it did open the possibility that it may still attempt to finalize and implement a permanent vaccine and testing mandate (Lewis &

Heidingfelder, 2022). In the meantime, occupational health nurses must monitor compliance with specific standards of care associated with best practices in COVID-19 care in a way that complies with the General Duty Clause. Under that clause, OSHA requires employers to provide a workplace "free from recognized hazards that are causing or are likely to cause death or serious physical harm" (29 C.F.R. 654). "Employers can be cited for violation of the General Duty Clause if a recognized serious hazard exists in their workplace and the employer does not take reasonable steps to prevent or abate the hazard. The General Duty Clause is used only where there is no standard that applies to the particular hazard" (Lewis & Heidingsfelder, 2022, p. 1). OSHA's most recent guidance from its National Emphasis Program (NEP) on COVID-19 recommends that employers implement the following:

- Facilitate employees getting vaccinated, including providing time off (paid or unpaid) to get vaccinated.
- Encourage workers who are infected or who have been exposed to stay home from work.
- Implement physical distancing for unvaccinated and at-risk workers.
- Provide face coverings or face masks for unvaccinated and at-risk workers.
- Educate and train workers on COVID-19 policies and procedures in languages they can understand.
- Suggest that unvaccinated guests wear face coverings in public-facing workplaces and that all guests wear face coverings in public, indoor settings in areas of substantial or high transmission (NEP).
- Maintain ventilation systems.
- Perform routine cleaning and disinfection.
- Record and report COVID-19 infections, hospitalizations, and deaths when applicable.
- Implement protections from retaliation and consider an anonymous process for voicing concerns related to COVID-19 (OSHA, 2021).
- Occupational health nurses should work with employers on designing, implementing, and evaluating programs that support these recommendations.

The Challenges of Providing Care for Rural Veterans

The U.S. rural and remote veteran population is ethnically, racially, and culturally diverse (Bushy, 2022). The Veterans Association (VA) (2023) documents 4.7 million rural and highly rural veterans, including 2.7 million enrolled in the VA have been impacted greatly by the social determinants of health, which the COVID-19 pandemic has exacerbated. Table 6.4 highlights the demographic impact of the physical, biopsychosocial, and technological barriers that veterans must overcome daily.

The occupational health nurse should inquire if and where a veteran served, as this information often provides insight into existing and potential diagnoses that might be exacerbated by COVID-19. "The older veteran population is more likely to be diagnosed with diabetes, obesity, high blood pressure, and heart conditions which often require frequent, ongoing, and costly care" (Bushy, 2022, p. 261). These conditions are also synonymous with life-threatening outcomes when these individuals are exposed to COVID-19. Therefore, the role of the occupational health nurse may range in scope from preventive education to direct patient care and long-term support services.

TABLE 6.4 Barriers to Rural Veteran Health Care

Challenge	Demographic	Impact of COVID-19
Access to care	There are 4.7 million highly rural veterans, but only 2.7 million are enrolled in the U.S. Department of Veterans Affairs (VA).	The long-term effect of the virus has contributed to increases in physical, mental health, and social concerns and further isolated this vulnerable population.
Service-connected comorbidities	Fifty-eight percent of rural enrolled veterans have at least one service-connected physical or behavioral health diagnosed condition.	The impact of COVID has been evidenced to worsen preexisting physical and behavioral health comorbidities.
Gender disparities	Eight percent of enrolled rural veterans are women.	Most female veterans who may be eligible for services related to COVID-19 are not connected to the VA system; therefore, these patients are at risk of being underserved.
Racial and ethnic disparities	Ten percent of enrolled rural veterans are minorities.	Occupational health nurses can lead initiatives that allow veterans from diverse backgrounds to access culturally competent care.
Financial challenges	Forty-four percent of rural U.S. veterans earn less than $35,000 annually.	The Office of Health Equity (OHE) worked with the National Center on Homelessness Among Veterans (NCHAV) to bring attention to the older homeless veterans population and the health disparities that exist in this group.
Technological barriers	Twenty-seven percent of rural U.S. veterans cannot access the internet at home.	The lack of internet connectivity further isolates rural veterans.
The aging of U.S. rural veterans	Rural veterans enrolled in the VA's health care system are significantly older: 55% are over the age of 65.	The need for access to comprehensive care for aging rural veterans suffering from complications related to COVID-19 is a mandate for the United States to expand communications and technologies so that health care can be delivered to veterans in rural areas throughout the United States.

Source: Table 6.4: Adapted from U.S. Department of Veterans Affairs, "Rural Veterans,"
https://www.ruralhealth.va.gov/aboutus/ruralvets.asp#vet.

Conclusion

Health care and governmental leaders have emphasized the vulnerability of rural communities since the beginning of the COVID-19 pandemic. Geographic, cultural, and economic barriers have made health care provisions daunting for rural health providers. These factors, along with the advanced age of many rural residents and the growing shortage of health care providers, have forced workers to leave the workforce and avoid care until they experience more advanced stages of chronic illnesses such as heart disease, diabetes, and various forms of cancer. The consequences of this behavior have placed rural residents at greater risk of contracting COVID-19 and increased the incidence of the virus in high-risk rural areas (Callaghan et al., 2021). The global nature of COVID-19 and its health consequences indicate that individuals and communities that understand these risks are more likely to engage in prevention strategies such as masking, social distancing, and vaccinations. This is when the role of the rural occupational health nurse becomes even more essential.

Although numerous studies have detailed the challenges nurses face in traditional acute and long-term care settings, less has been discussed regarding nursing practice in rural communities, particularly those communities where occupational health nurses may be the only providers of health services for hundreds of miles. The rural nurse may be the only connection a migrant or seasonal farm worker has within the health care system, despite the nurse having limited time to interact with a patient with multi-complex health concerns related to the long-term consequences of COVID-19. Before the COVID-19 pandemic, nurses focused on prevention techniques to protect workers from work-related injuries and illnesses. Additionally, nurses reviewed medications with patients and how they could access them for a long-term supply of vital drugs if their access was blocked by weather, natural disaster, or relocation. Since the onset of the pandemic, the focus of care for these nurses has expanded to teach the proper use of PPE to minimize the spread of the virus to family members and fellow workers. Additionally, using mobile clinics to reach those further removed from communication has allowed for vaccination clinics on wheels and the provision of care after work hours and when workers are resting (Moyce, 2022).

Perhaps one of the most valuable lessons from the COVID-19 pandemic is the need for nursing leaders to prioritize the mobility of nursing care as we approach a future that will most certainly include living with the COVID-19 virus. Three years into the COVID-19 pandemic, many occupational health rural nurses have returned to their clinical positions, providing compassionate, skilled care and advocacy for migrant and seasonal farm workers during and beyond regularly scheduled clinic hours. Nurses assist patients in accessing both appointments and access to those appointments, which increases the probability that workers will keep their scheduled appointments. Additionally, these nurses often arrange translation or interpreter services for patients with little or no English-speaking skills. Lastly, occupational health nurses are skilled in arranging wraparound services to meet patients' needs in one location (Moyce, 2022).

These nurse specialists continue to provide care and education in industrial, agricultural, school, and other community settings with minimal resources and personnel. Additionally, rural occupational health nurses provide educational support for those individuals who either do not trust experts or do not have access to care. Future priorities must include the creation of public policy initiatives that support rural occupational health nurses to create and lead collaborations with their urban colleagues in creating infrastructure supports to meet the needs of individuals, families, and the rural workforce as the virus continues to evolve.

Questions for Discussion Related to Case Study 6.1

1. What role could an occupational health nurse play in Javier's care? What are the priorities of care that must be addressed to meet Javier's needs?
2. What resources are available to migrant workers such as Javier? Consider resources to meet Javier's physical and psychosocial needs.

References

AgriSafe. (2022). *About us.* https://www.agrisafe.org/about/

Ávila, A. (2021). Essential or expendable during the COVID-19 pandemic? A student-lived experience on grieving the unjust and early deaths of vulnerable populations. *American Journal of Public Health, 111*(1), 66–68. https://doi.org/10.2105/AJPH.2020.306001

Birrell, A. (2022). *Respiratory protection has never been more important: Selection and considerations for proper use.* Occupational Health & Safety. https://ohsonline.com/Articles/2022/02/01/Respiratory-Protection-has-Never-Been-More-Important.aspx

Boles, S. (2020). *Coal and COVID-19: Lung impairment makes miners especially vulnerable to coronavirus.* Energy & Environment Health. https://ohiovalleyresource.org/2020/05/04/coal-and-covid-19-lung-impairment-makes-miners-especially-vulnerable-to-coronavirus/

Bushy, A. (2022). Rural veterans: Implications for nursing practice. In L.F. Ferguson & K. Lowrance (Eds.), *Rural health nursing: Barriers and Benefits.* (pp. 257-271). DEStech Publications, Inc.

Bushy, A. (2000). *Orientation to Nursing in the Rural Community.* SAGE Publications, Incorporated. https://doi.org/10.4135/9781452204871

Callaghan, T., Lueck, J. A., Trujillo, K. L., & Ferdinand, A. O. (2021). Rural and urban differences in COVID-19 prevention behaviors. *The Journal of Rural Health, 37*(2), 287–295. https://doi.org/10.1111/jrh.12556

Clement, J., Jacobi, M., & Greenwood, B. N. (2021). Patient access to chronic medications during the Covid-19 pandemic: Evidence from a comprehensive dataset of US insurance claims. *PloS One, 16*(4), e0249453.https://doi.org/10.1371/journal.pone.0249453

Clemmons-Brown, C. A. (2020). Addressing human trafficking through nurse leadership: Application of AONL competencies. *Nurse Leader, 18*(6), 581–585. https://doi.org/10.1016/j.mnl.2020.01.005

Constantin, J., Ullrich, F., & Mueller, K. J. (2022). *Rural and urban pharmacy presence— Pharmacy deserts.* Rural Policy Research Institute. https://rupri.public-health.uiowa.edu/publications/policybriefs/2022/Pharmacy%20Deserts.pdf

Cybersecurity and Infrastructure Security Agency, U.S. Department of Homeland Security. (2021). *Guidance on the essential critical infrastructure workforce.* https://www.cisa.gov/publication/guidance-essential-critical-infrastructure-workforce

Fahs, P. (2020). COVID-19 and rural healthcare. *Online Journal of Rural Nursing and Health Care, 20*(1), 1–2.

Gomez, J. (2020, June 7). *COVID-19 rapidly spreading in a town of migrant workers who can't afford to stay home.* Matter of Fact. https://www.matteroffact.tv/covid-19-rapidly-spreading-in-a-town-of-migrant-workers-who-cant-afford-to-stay-home/

Gomez, J. (2021, January 10). *A town of migrant workers who can't afford to stay home.* Matter of Fact. https://www.matteroffact.tv/a-town-of-migrant-workers-who-cant-afford-to-stay-home/

International Labour Organizations. (2022). *ILO declaration of fundamental principles and right at work and its follow-up.* https://www.ilo.org/wcmsp5/groups/public/---ed_norm/---declaration/documents/normativeinstrument/wcms_716594.pdf

Lewis, S., & Heidingsfelder, J. (2022). *Life after OSHA withdraws vaccine mandate.* Occupational Health & Safety. https://ohsonline.com/articles/2022/02/03/life-after-osha-withdraws-vaccine-mandate.aspx?admgarea=covid19

Lusk, J. L., & Chandra, R. (2021). Farmer and farm worker illnesses and deaths from COVID-19 and impacts on agricultural output. *PloS One, 16*(4), e0250621.https://doi.org/10.1371/journal.pone.0250621

Moyce, S. (2022). Risks to safety and health for migrant and seasonal farmworkers. In C. A. Winters (Ed.), *Rural nursing: Concepts, theory, and practice* (6th ed., 337–348). Springer.

National Center for Farmworker Health. (2022, January). *Facts about farmworkers*. https://www.ncfh.org/uploads/3/8/6/8/38685499/facts_about_farmworkers_fact_sheet_1.10.23.pdf

National Human Trafficking Hotline. (2024). https://humantraffickinghotline.org/en/human-trafficking

Nease, D., Tamez, M., Barrientos-Ortiz, C., Fisher, M., Brewer, S., & Zittleman, L. (2022). 150 engagement to reduce COVID-19 vaccine hesitancy—The value of investments in long term community relationships. *Journal of Clinical and Translational Science, 6*(s1), 14–15. https://doi.org/10.1017/cts.2022.60

Occupational Safety and Health Administration. (2021). *OSHA direction*. https://www.osha.gov/sites/default/files/enforcement/directives/DIR_2021-03_CPL_03.pdf

Peters, D. J. (2020). Community susceptibility and resiliency to COVID-19 across the rural-urban continuum in the United States. *The Journal of Rural Health, 36*(3), 446–456. https://doi.org/10.1111/jrh.12477

Raker, K. A. (2020). Human trafficking education: A guide for nurse educators. *Journal of Professional Nursing, 36*(6), 692–697. https://doi.org/10.1016/j.profnurs.2020.09.015

Tate, R. A. (2020). *COVID-19 cases on the rise in coal mines: New outbreaks expose health risks of underground coal mining, lack of transparency in public data*. Global Energy Monitor. https://globalenergymonitor.org/wp-content/uploads/2021/01/Briefing_-Coal-Mines-and-COVID-19-June-2020.pdf

U.S. Department of Homeland Security. (n.d.). *What is human trafficking?* https://www.dhs.gov/blue-campaign/what-human-trafficking

U.S. Department of Veterans Affairs. (2023, June 23). *Rural veterans*. https://www.ruralhealth.va.gov/aboutus/ruralvets.asp#vet

Van Dorn, A., Cooney, R. E., & Sabin, M. L. (2020). COVID-19 exacerbating inequalities in the US. *The Lancet, 395*(10232), 1243–1244. https://doi.org/10.1016/S0140-6736(20)30893-X

Wade, W. (2020). *USA: Coal miners' union warns that members face heightened risk of exposure and complications from Covid-19*. Business & Human Rights Resource Center. https://www.business-humanrights.org/en/latest-news/usa-coal-miners-union-warns-that-members-face-heightened-risk-of-exposure-and-complications-from-covid-19

World Health Organization. (2022). *Occupational health: health workers*. https://www.who.int/news-room/fact-sheets/detail/occupational-health--health-workers

Image Credits

CHAPTER 7

Providing Telehealth for Specialty Care

The COVID-19 pandemic was initially reported in December 2019 and was declared such by the World Health Organization (WHO) on March 11, 2020 (Pujolar et al., 2022). The world was not prepared for the COVID-19 virus at the beginning of the pandemic, which started in China and quickly moved to other parts of the world. While the pandemic started in 2019, it was predicted to arrive in northeastern United States in March of 2020. In the late winter of 2020, public health specialists coordinated to open one of the first ambulatory care clinics in Massachusetts to care for what was predicted to be the first surge of patients. Cohen et al. (2020) stated that the initial challenges during those first weeks included discovering commonalities in the patterns of patient symptoms since physical exams were often limited due to many patients' reluctance to seek medical care. A second challenge for health care providers was discerning what might be symptoms of the COVID-19 virus and influenza since the symptomatology and severity varied widely among the patient population. One early symptom of COVID was loss of smell, which many patients reported during the first few days of the illness. Most patients recovered from their symptoms in 2 to 3 weeks; however, there were some patients who experienced dyspnea (shortness of breath) between day 4 and day 10 (Cohen et al., 2020). Additionally, providers were challenged by an unprecedented sense of fear and anxiety among community members who were understandably fearful that a diagnosis of COVID-19 was in fact a death sentence.

COVID-19 Impact on the Public's Health

The COVID-19 pandemic and the public health measures taken had a profound effect on health care in the United States and beyond, including on public health and the economy. Some strategies that were taken to combat the rapidly increasing number of COVID-19 cases negatively affected access to health care and patient acute and chronic conditions. Initially, the classification of services as essential and nonessential allowed resources to be redirected to the pandemic response. This redirection led to cancellations or delays in elective and nonurgent procedures. Second, social distancing was required to reduce interactions between people. Included in social distancing was partial or complete lockdowns of schools and nonessential businesses, with instructions to stay at home, which became a barrier to seeking health care. Due to a misinterpretation of government recommendations, many did not seek health services for fear of contracting the virus, believing they would have difficulties in gaining health care access or that the services were of poor quality, as well as the stigma of receiving a COVID-19 diagnosis. The lack of materials and medical supplies also contributed to increasing negative perceptions of the quality of the health services, especially in disadvantaged settings or situations with structural difficulties.

An indirect effect of the pandemic was on the U.S. economy. There was a rise in unemployment, a loss of household income that resulted in loss of insurance coverage and thus health care access, difficulties in making copayments, and difficulty obtaining transportation to appointments and homelessness (Pujolar et al., 2022). While all Americans were impacted by the economic crisis, vulnerable populations suffered a greater impact. Individuals with low socioeconomic status, the elderly, chronically ill patients or those with severe health conditions, migrants from countries that are low income, and rural residents experienced indirect negative effects related to health care access and the quality of curative and preventive care provided for other conditions, as well as the exacerbation of difficulties and barriers related to socioeconomic factors (Pujolar et al., 2022).

All of this added significant disruption to health care provision, resulting in a decrease in the use of services during the initial onset of the pandemic and with the onset of new COVID-19 waves. After the first few months and progressive COVID waves, there was an increase in the utilization of services; however, levels did not reach prepandemic levels, resulting in individuals with cancer, heart disease, and other acute conditions needing treatment presenting with advanced stages and morbidities.

Clinic Care

Primary care clinics in the United States saw a drop in the number of in-person visits and an increase in remote care consultations. The use of online consultation increased during the pandemic to address the difficulties in access. However, this increased the inequalities to access to care and further isolated marginal community members. Individuals reported access problems related to a lack of understanding of digital devices or lack of internet connection or mobile devices. Additionally, there was a perception that the care received in virtual consultation was impersonal.

COVID-19 had a large impact on outpatient primary care offices affiliated with hospitals. To cover the needs of the hospital due to the influx of critically ill patients, providers were moved from outpatient clinics to acute care settings. One hospital in the New England area found themselves in this situation. Their ambulatory clinics cared for over 40,000 active patients a year, with most insured through a state-funded insurance program. To cover the acute care areas, these clinics ran with a skeleton crew that was required to maintain social distancing, resulting in a transformation of how they cared for patients which restricted routine visits (Doolittle et al., 2020). Through the implementation of a new communication model, they transitioned more than 400 daily visits to telehealth. However, the transition to telehealth, while effective, was not without challenges. There was an inequity of resources with many patients not having access to computers, leading to visits occurring via telephone. Unfortunately, due to regulatory barriers the use of telephone visits was not an approved telehealth platform. Despite these regulatory limitations, the ambulatory clinic was able to reach 70% of their pre-COVID patients (Doolittle et al., 2020).

Prior to the pandemic, the use of telehealth was being explored by some clinics, "approximately 61% of healthcare institutions and 40%-50% of all hospitals in the United States used some form of telehealth" (Luna et al., 2022, p. 2). Early adopters of telehealth appreciated the low cost, ability to monitor patients with chronic diseases, time and workforce utilized more effectively and easy patient access. However, universal use was limited due to technical barriers and "regulatory, financial, and health system challenges" (Luna et al., 2022, p. 2). The Centers for Medicare and Medicaid (CMS) initiated enhanced reimbursement for these types of visits as well as increasing broadband across predominantly rural states, with federal funding to support this method of care. As of May 2020, all states cover primary care services through Medicaid, with some states approving reimbursement for telephone services in September 2021 (Luna et al., 2022) making telehealth became a viable option for many outpatient clinics.

Many clinics and providers expressed satisfaction with telehealth, but there were some areas that patients appreciated about face-to-face care. In a study conducted by Luna et al. (2022) to elicit how patients felt about telehealth visits, patients responded that they received care from multiple ambulatory settings, including internal medicine, hematology–oncology, cardiology, primary care, and endocrinology, which was different than prepandemic areas (Figure 7.1).

Overall, patients had positive experiences using telehealth. Many patients who used telehealth found the video and audio quality were good and felt the instructions before the visit were useful. Almost 90% of patients agreed the quality of care they received was good and that they were interested in future telehealth visits. Nearly half of the patients surveyed reported saving 1 hour of travel time, 10.4% saved 2 to 4 hours, and 2.4% saved over 4 hours. They noted "a positive correlation between satisfaction with quality of care received, satisfaction with the ease of using the telehealth application, ratings for video and audio quality, ratings for instructions before the visit, and time saved" (Luna et al., 2022, p. 3). Because patients were satisfied with telehealth, maintaining future telehealth use, and improving the patient experience, the quality of telehealth delivery platforms and instructions provided to patients must be enhanced and improved.

CASE STUDY 7.1

Jane cares for her elderly father (Ralph), which includes taking him to his medical appointments with his internal medicine provider. Ralph's internal medicine provider is located at the nearest medical center, which is an hour commute each way. The trip is hard for both Jane and Ralph as Ralph is not very mobile and has chronic pain. At the start of the pandemic Ralph's provider informed them that his visits would be held via telehealth over the computer due to state and government regulations. They were happy that they would not have to make the trip; however, while they owned a computer, they did not have internet access as they live in a remote area. Jane contacted the provider's office to explain the situation and they agreed to conduct Ralph's visit over the phone.

Oncology

Some specialty clinics worldwide also experienced changes in their levels of activity, such as oncology, maternal health, and mental health. The challenges illuminated the need for drastic changes in infrastructure to meet the needs of patients living with oncology diagnoses

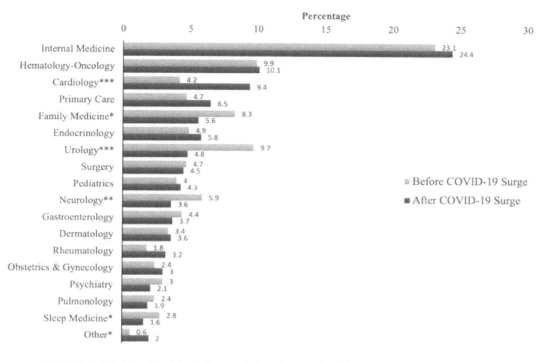

FIGURE 7.1 Telehealth visits before and after the pandemic by specialty.

that required emergent interventions. Yackzan and Shah (2021) stated that oncology nurses have led initiatives to address the needs of persons living with oncology diagnoses, including access to care and services throughout the ongoing pandemic. Multimodal screenings became the norm in these settings. The increased practice of pre-appointment screening calls along with onsite screenings serve to support the public health recommendations and ease the fears of patients who are most at risk for exposure to the COVID-19 virus.

Telemedicine, which was still in relative infancy when the pandemic hit, exploded overnight, with telehealth visits growing exponentially. To ensure access to care for patients, many clinics transitioned to telehealth visits. COVID-19 had a broad impact on oncology patient care, which included the rapid adoption of telehealth visits (Thomas et al., 2022). In one oncology practice on the West Coast, the proportion of telehealth visits increased during the beginning of March 2020 (Thomas et al., 2022), from 0.6% to 87% in the first 3 weeks of March 2020; in-person visits decreased from 98% to 3%.

Maternal Health

Maternal health is critical for the health of the child. However, health care equity for individuals in rural and underserved areas has been a longtime struggle. Less than one half of the women living in rural America are within a 30-minute drive to obstetric services (Health Resources and Services Administration [HRSA], 2023), with more than 10% needing to drive 100 or more miles for care. Telehealth is one way to bridge this gap. Telehealth can address multiple barriers for maternal health, including routine prenatal and postnatal care, for

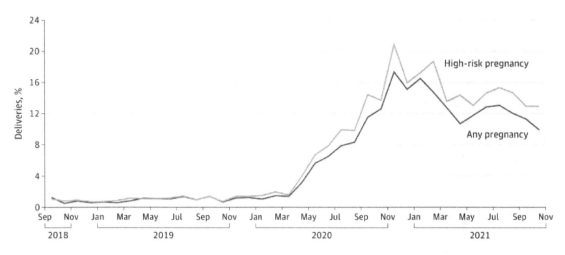

FIGURE 7.2   Percentage of deliveries each month with prenatal telehealth visits during 40-week pregnancy period.

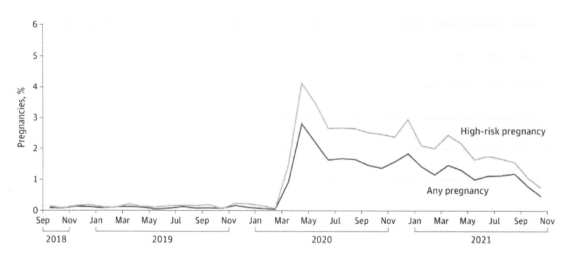

FIGURE 7.3   Percentage of pregnancies each month with prenatal telehealth visits.

patients who do not have the ability to travel to a health care provider. Additionally, telehealth offers more choices of providers for patients of color (Figures 7.2 and 7.3).

In May 2020, the Maternal Telehealth Access Project was funded for 1 year by the Coronavirus Aid, Relief and Economic Security Act (CARES Act) to increase access to quality maternity care and services via telehealth for women of color. The project focused on caring for women at the greatest risk of maternal mortality and morbidity: Black women, Native American women, Latinx women, and women who live in rural and frontier communities. This is important as maternal mortality impacts women of color at higher rates, and the pandemic made this disparity worse. Data from the CDC demonstrated that COVID-19 mortality rates are substantially higher among Black and Latinx women. Women of color had also expressed concern about how they can safely obtain prenatal care, deliver their babies, feed their babies, and receive needed postpartum support services, including mental health care. The Maternal Telehealth Access Project (Maternal Health Learning & Innovation Center, 2023) sought to address these concerns while supporting providers and families with access to telehealth and distant care services.

In addition to routine maternal health services, telehealth can offer screenings for antepartum and postpartum complications that require immediate attention such as pre-eclampsia, postpartum depression, and infection. Even with the advantage of telehealth visits for maternal health patients, there are limitations. Patients do need to present to a clinic for visits requiring internal exams, diagnosis and treatment for severe illness, and treatment. Through partial funding from the HRSA, the Rural Obstetrics (OB) Access and Maternal Services network (ROAMS, 2023) provides telehealth obstetric care to rural northeastern New Mexico. ROAMS's network provides services with the goal of reducing maternal mortality and improving OB access. ROAMS connects expecting parents with OB services and maternal-fetal medicine specialists who do not have OB services available in their area. In addition to typical telehealth visits, patients are provided with home telehealth kits that automatically send medical data, such as blood pressure and blood glucose levels, directly to the physicians monitoring their pregnancy.

Prenatal telehealth visits increased substantially during the early phase of the COVID-19 pandemic, with the highest percentage occurring in April 2020 (Acharya et al., 2023). Acharya et al. (2023) conducted a study to identify the trends in telehealth visits from 2018 to 2021. While their study sample included mostly commercially insured patients, it does bring to light the trends in OB telehealth visits. The highest number of pregnant patients utilizing telehealth services were pregnant patients with anxiety and depression.

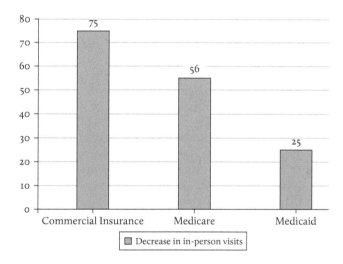

FIGURE 7.4 Percentage of decrease in in-person behavioral health visits by insurance.

Conclusion

The pandemic impacted all aspects of health care. In this chapter we discussed the changes made to ambulatory care. At the beginning of the pandemic, there was a drop in the number of patients presenting to ambulatory clinics due to government and state mandates and the fear of contracting the virus. Telehealth became an alternative to receiving health care in primary care and specialty clinics (Figure 7.4). Telemedicine, which was still in relative infancy when the pandemic hit, exploded overnight, with telehealth visits growing exponentially. COVID-19 had a broad impact on all patients, including the rapid adoption of telehealth visits. Now that the pandemic is resolving, there have been changes to how patients receive health care and to reimbursement for telehealth visits.

Questions for Discussion Related to Case Study 7.1

1. What are the limitations to a medical appointment via telephone? Would the limitation be the same via teleconferencing?
2. Would having remote medical appointments affect Ralph's health care?
3. What are the advantages to telehealth for Ralph and Jane? For the provider?

References

Acharya, M., Ali, M. M., Hayes, C. J., Bogulski, C. A., Magann, E. F., & Eswaran, H. (2023). Trends in telehealth visits during pregnancy, 2018 to 2021. *JAMA Network Open*, 6(4), e236630. https://doi.org/10.1001/jamanetworkopen.2023.6630

Cohen, P. A., Hall, L.E., John, J. N., & Rapoport, A. B. (2020). The early natural history of SARS-CoV-2 infection: Clinical observations from an urban, ambulatory COVID-19 clinic. *Mayo Clin Proc*, 95(6) 1124–1126. https://doi.org/10.1016/j.mayocp.2020.04.010

Doolittle, B. R., Richards, B., Tarabar, A., Ellman, M., & Tobin, D. (2020). The day the residents left: Lessons learnt from COVID-19 for ambulatory clinics. *Family Medical Community Health*, 8(3), e000513. https://doi.org/10.1136/fmch-2020-000513

Health Resources and Services Administration. (2023). *Best practice guide: Telehealth for maternal health services*. https://telehealth.hhs.gov/providers/best-practice-guides/ telehealth-for-maternal-health-services/bridging-the-gaps-with-telehealth

Luna. P., Lee, M., Greeno, R. V., DeLucia, N., London, Y., Hoffman, P., Burg, M., Harris, K, Spatz, E. S., Mena-Hurtado, C., & Smolderen, K.G. (2022). Telehealth care before and during COVID-19: Trends and quality in a large health system. *JAMIA Open*, 5(4), 1–9. https://www.ncbi.nlm.nih.gov/pmc/articles/PMC9531686/pdf/ooac079.pdf

Maternal Health Learning & Innovation Center. (2023). *Maternal Telehealth Access Project*. https://maternalhealthlearning.org/telehealth/

Pujolar, G., Oliver-Anglès, A., Vargas, I., & Vázquez, M. (2022). Changes in access to health services during the COVID-19 pandemic: A scoping review. *International Journal of Environmental Research and Public Health*, 19, 1749. https:// doi.org/10.3390/ijerph19031749

Rural OB Access and Maternal Services. (2023). *Home page*. https://roamsnm.org

Thomas, T., Nobrega, J. C., & Britton-Susino, S. (2022). Challenges and collaborations: A case study for successful sexual assault nurse examiner education in rural communities during the COVID-19 pandemic. *Journal of Forensic Nursing*, 18(1), 59–63.

Yackzan, S., & Shah, M. (2021). Ambulatory oncology: Infrastructure development in response to the COVID-19 pandemic. *Clinical Journal of Oncology Nursing*, 25(1), 41–47.

Image Credits

UNIT IV

Impact on Mental Health

Before and during the pandemic, behavioral mental health care had been both a challenge and an opportunity. The pandemic exacerbated the need for both behavioral mental health services and services for individuals with both mental health and substance use disorders. Due to the needs for these types of services and increased barriers to care, there was an increase in telehealth behavioral mental health services.

Prior to the pandemic, the demand for behavioral health services was increasing. In 2019, it was estimated that 52 million adults in the United States reported having a mental, behavioral, or emotional disorder (American Hospital Association [AHA], 2022). Additionally, 20 million individuals aged 12 or older reported having a substance use disorder, which included alcohol abuse, illicit drug abuse, or both (AHA, 2022). Since the start of the pandemic, there has been a three-fold increase in the number of individuals reporting symptoms of anxiety or depression. The number of individuals reporting suicidal ideation has also increased three-fold, and annual drug overdoses have increased by 30%. Even with the increase in services there were other barriers such as limited number of providers, loss of health care coverage, stay-at-home mandates, and patients generally avoiding care due to COVID-19 concerns (AHA, 2022). This resulted in a decrease of in-person outpatient behavioral health visits.

Reference

American Hospital Association. (2022). *TrendWatch: The impacts of the COVID-19 pandemic on behavioral health*. https://www.aha.org/system/files/media/file/2022/05/trendwatch-the-impacts-of-the-covid-19-pandemic-on-behavioral-health.pdf

CHAPTER 8

Mental Health Effect of Health Care Providers

The pandemic had a profound effect on the health care workforce. Health care workers suffered both physical and emotional strain from treating COVID-19 patients (Figure 8.1). Health care workers on the frontlines of the pandemic were at risk due to daily exposure to patients with COVID and lack of adequate PPE. The pandemic impacted their mental health and contributed to anxiety, stress, depression, and loneliness. The stress led to sleep disturbances, headaches, stomachaches, and increased drug and alcohol use. Yet only 13% of frontline workers received behavioral health services due to worry and stress (AHA, 2022).

The COVID-19 pandemic placed health care workers under psychological stress. The prevalence of mental health disorders was determined in a systematic review of 20 studies with 10,886 health care workers from across China (Hao et al., 2021). Female health care workers and nurses had a higher prevalence of depression and anxiety, with frontline workers having the highest incidence of anxiety. In their analysis, Hao et al. (2021) concluded depression was noted in 14 of the 20 studies included in the analysis, with the prevalence of depressive symptoms among all health care workers at 24.1%, the percentage of secondline health care workers at 36.2%, and female health care workers at 38.6%. Frontline health care workers (14.6%) experienced moderate to severe depression. Anxiety was also prevalent. Sixteen of the studies offered the prevalence of anxiety symptoms among all health care at 28.6% (Hao et al., 2021). Frontline health care providers had a higher prevalence of anxiety (33.5%) than secondline health care workers (Hao et al., 2021). Female health care workers experienced a higher level of anxiety than their male counterparts at 26.6%. Just over 44% reported anxiety, with 11.8% reporting moderate to severe anxiety (Hao et al., 2021). Posttraumatic stress disorder (PTSD) has been noted as a sequela of the pandemic. Hao et al. (2021) reported a prevalence of PTSD among 25.6% of health care workers.

Rural nurses may be at greater risk for PTSD with increased exposure to traumatic incidents in the workplace (Lenthall et al., 2019). Rural nurses can be more vulnerable to traumatic events due to caring for a wide variety of individuals living in sparsely populated areas, with many residents working in high-risk occupations (Jahner et al., 2019). This is compounded by living

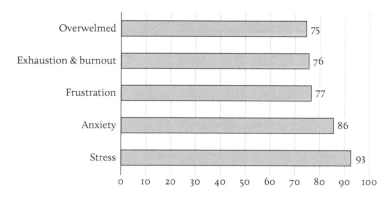

FIGURE 8.1 Percentage of health care workers experiencing mental health symptoms.

and working in the same community as family members and friends, leading to limited anonymity and blurring of personal and professional boundaries. When there is a connection between the caregiver, the nurse, and a patient's traumatic experience, especially a patient the nurse is familiar with, the nurse may experience symptoms of PTSD (Jahner et al., 2019).

Terry et al. (2015) found that workplace health and safety was challenging in rural and remote areas where death and tragedy are common, and burnout or compassion fatigue are seldom identified as areas of concern. Rural and remote nurses' experience of distressing events may be complicated in communities where their work and personal lives are intertwined. Rural and remote nurses frequently deal with injury and death of people they personally know, and they work in isolation and have limited access to trauma-response teams or advanced care services (Jahner et al., 2020). In addition, rural and remote nurses need to be aware of the safety of their patients and themselves. In rural settings there are often limited or no on-site security or police backup when nurses encounter an aggressive or violent patient or family member (Jahner et al., 2020).

Rural nurses were surveyed to understand their experiences of distressing incidents, with three main themes identified (Jahner et al., 2020). The first was involvement in profound events of death/dying, traumatic injury, and loss, with some nurses highlighting intense emotional pain and anxiety as well as difficulty in processing the events. The nurses focused on the total volume of experiences over time and "a sense of feeling powerlessness, especially when caring for people with whom they had a relationship within the community" (Jahner et al., 2020, p. 483).

The second theme that emerged was experiencing or witnessing severe violence and/ or aggression. The nurses reported feelings of distress when caring for victims of interpersonal violence in cases of spousal and elder abuse. They also reported feelings of "extreme anguish/sorrow when dealing with neglect, physical abuse, sexual assault, or violence directed toward children" (Jahner et al., 2020, p. 483).

The final theme was failure to rescue or protect patients or clients. Many of the nurses experienced distress when they were not able to rescue or protect patients under their care. The nurses reported delayed or inadequate response times, emergent situations with complications, and deficient equipment or equipment failure that negatively influenced patient outcomes. Nurses are with patients more hours than other health care providers, so nurses commonly notice deteriorating situations that require interventions. Some nurses who responded to the survey "described unsuccessful attempts to escalate physician intervention and responsiveness after a sudden change in a patient's health status, or dismissal of their attempt to achieve a patient transfer to a more advanced care facility" (Jahner et al., 2020, p. 483). This left many nurses overwhelmed with self-blame and shame.

Each of the themes has a large impact on the nurse and the nurse's mental health. The nurses felt like they were well supported in the work setting with debriefing and informal peer support (Jahner et al., 2020). Some of the organizations offered formal debriefing and provided opportunities to access mental health services. However, some organizations demonstrated a lack of acknowledgement or support, downplaying the events (Jahner et al., 2020). This led to a lack of timely and appropriate follow-up, including their need for safety.

Health Care Workers' Access to Services

There were barriers for rural and remote nurses to adequate mental health services. Support was slow and inadequate (Jahner et al., 2020). Some nurses were instructed to contact their Employee and Family Assistance Program (EFAP); however, they experienced inconsistent availability. Living in a rural area with close community ties prevented some nurses from disclosing the details of their experiences and violating the Health Insurance Portability and Accountability Act (HIPAA). Some nurses preferred to remain private while others "did not seek support given their personal ties to the community, issues of confidentiality, concerns for their own reputation, or their sense of professional obligation to deal with it on their own, or you are expected to suck it up and get back to work" (Jahner et al., 2020, p. 487).

Pandemic's Impact on Health Care Worker's Health

The pandemic also impacted health care workers' sleep patterns (Hao et al., 2021). A considerable number of health care workers experienced sleep disturbances during the pandemic, with an estimate that two in five were affected (Pappa et al., 2021). Poor quality of sleep can impact cognitive function and decision-making, leading to a reduction in work efficiency and an increase in medical errors (Pappa et al., 2021). Lack of sleep has an impact not only mental health but also physical health. Poor sleep is related to obesity, diabetes, heart attack, and stroke and has been associated with increased probability of respiratory illnesses such as the common cold and pneumonia (Pappa et al., 2021).

This was even more acute in rural settings where many health care providers did not feel comfortable acknowledging their anxiety and depression in small communities where everyone knows everyone else. The patients they cared for presented with highly complex needs and there were few or no resources to provide for these clients (MacLeod et al., 2022), which added frustration for the health care provider. Despite the apparent potential for intervention to maintain a healthy workforce, the consistent message from many is that health care systems did not address their needs. Many health care providers suffered tantamount stress as a result of very sick patients and family members who did not believe the virus to be real, the fear of becoming infected themselves, exposure of family and friends, fear of losing employment related to decreased number of patients being treated in ambulatory settings, or short staffing resulting in working many days with no time off. The provision of mental health care for health care workers was not a priority, and many did not feel comfortable asking for help with their mental health concerns. The WHO (2022) indicated that as many as 23% to 46% of health care professionals expressed symptoms of anxiety while 20%–37% experienced depression during the COVID-19 pandemic.

Critical care nurses and doctors experienced the most exposure to the virus. Many of these professionals were aware of their vulnerability to both the virus itself but also the emotional toll from such high death rates. A study by Crow et al. (2020), showed 56.9% of participants had depression, 67% reported anxiety, and 54.1% stress after the first wave of COVID-19. Nurses working in rural health care settings have always identified the stress and anxiety they have from the responsibilities that they must care for family and friends, something that is unique to rural health care. However, the pandemic added feelings of frustration related to misinformation and ethical dilemmas that ranged from knowledge of community members who tested positive for COVID-19 to resource allocation to administrative response. As noted by Alexander (2021), "If you view our occupation through a capitalistic lens, as it's so obvious most health care management does, because since 2016, the average hospital turned over 83% of their RN workforce, due to a combination of churn and burn at the lower end of the experience scale, and older RNs retiring out. Those of us sandwiched in the middle, trying to hold down the fort, are dying" (p. 350).

Conclusion

The COVID-19 pandemic changed health care systems throughout the world. Nurses were forced to work long hours, leading to physical discomfort and extreme exhaustion, all while fearing contagion and emotional distress. These high levels of stress lead to behavioral and psychiatric disorders, including depression, anxiety, insomnia, psychological distress, and posttraumatic stress among nurses. Unfortunately, these symptoms have not returned to prepandemic levels. On a scale of 1 to 10, with 10 being the most positive and 1 being the most negative, nurses surveyed in the 2022 frontline nurse mental health & wellbeing survey (Trusted Health, 2022) rated their current mental health and well-being at an average of 5.8; this is a decrease from the prepandemic levels of 7.8 (Figure 8.2). While the previous year's studies found a slight decrease from 29% to 28%, this demonstrates that even while the acute phase of the pandemic has subsided, nurses continue to feel lasting mental health effects.

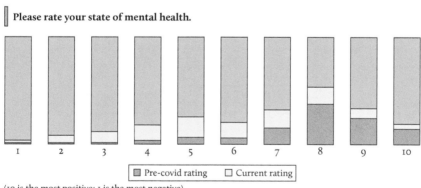

Please rate your state of mental health.

1 2 3 4 5 6 7 8 9 10

☐ Pre-covid rating ☐ Current rating

(10 is the most positive; 1 is the most negative)

FIGURE 8.2 Nurses' mental health has not rebounded to its prepandemic levels.

The negative effects on nurses' physical and mental health because of the pandemic continue to be of concern. Most of the nurses reported (Trusted Health, 2022; Figure 8.3) the following:

- feelings of burnout (75%)
- compassion fatigue (66%)
- depression (64%)

Since the COVID-19 pandemic began, which of the following statements apply to you?

75%	I've experienced burnout
66%	I've experienced compassion fatigue towards my patients
64%	I've experienced feelings of depression
64%	My physical health has declined
50%	I've experienced feelings of trauma, extreme stress and/or ptsd
50%	I've been verbally attacked, intimidated or assaulted by a patient or his/her family
46%	I've experienced a moral injury or similar feelings related to ethical dilemmas such as rationing patient care
22%	I've been physically attacked, intimidated or assaulted by a patient or his/her family
10%	I've had suicidal thoughts

FIGURE 8.3 The negative effects on nurses' physical and mental health.

- decline in physical health (64%)
- extreme feeling of trauma, extreme stress, and/or PTSD (50%)

Mental health support can come from nurses' employers. More than half the nurses in the survey reported they were dissatisfied with the support their faculty provided them related to their mental health and well-being (Figure 8.4).

How satisfied are you with the level of support your current facility provides related to your mental health and well-being?

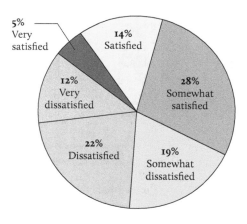

FIGURE 8.4 Nurses' satisfaction of support from current facility related to their mental health and well-being.

While over 50% of the respondents did not feel supported by their current facility, nearly 60% said that they were "very unlikely" or "somewhat unlikely" to share their thoughts or mental health concerns with a manager or individual at their facility (Figure 8.5). When

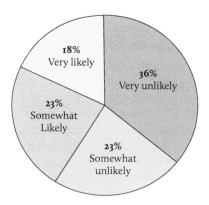

If you were experiencing acute depression, suicidal thoughts or mental health issues that you felt could negatively impact your ability to perform your job, how likely would you be to share this with your manager or other individual at your facility?

FIGURE 8.5 Nurses unlikely to seek support at work.

asked about the reasons for not seeking support, the leading reasons included (Trusted Health, 2022) the following:

- concerns of confidentiality (74%)
- concerns about job security (68%)
- concern there would be no effort to address the issue (64%)
- concern about potential impact on nursing license (44%)

While many of the nurses surveyed reported they would not seek treatment through their current facility, 40% did not know what mental health benefits their current facility offered (Figure 8.6).

Which of the following benefits does your current facility offer?
Which of the following benefits would you find most beneficial?

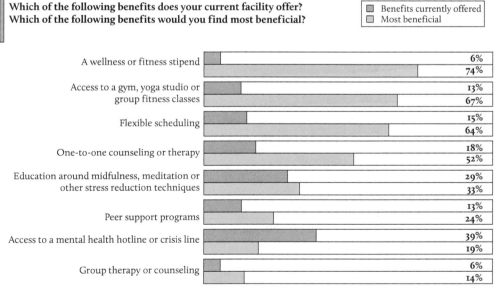

FIGURE 8.6 What benefits does your current facility offer?

There is no debate the COVID pandemic had an impact on nursing as a whole and on each individual nurse. One of the positive aspects that came from the pandemic was that nurses learned how to cluster and to be more effective in their care. Nurses became more intentional in their interactions; they were accustomed to going in and out of patient rooms and not actually taking time to spend with patients. Charity stated that one change as a result of COVID is that she no longer feels that she has to balance everything, always trying to give everybody equal amounts of time. The way she delivers patient care has changed; she doesn't know if this change is a bad thing, but it bothers her sometimes that she doesn't take as much time with the person/patient who is just having a normal bad day. Charity admits that she is not the same nurse she was before COVID: "I'm not going to lie; I still have a black box. I'm dealing with it slowly. I bring it out every day, but there are little parts of it that just are hard."

Questions for Discussion Related to Case Study 8.1

1. Is resilience a quality based on nature or nurture? What obligations (if any) do rural health care leaders have to provide educational and emotional supports to maintain and enhance resilience for nursing and health care staff?
2. Can resilience be reestablished following a prolonged, traumatic event? Describe strategies that nursing and health care leaders could implement to reignite both resilience and grit in frontline staff who provided care during the height of the COVID-19 pandemic.
3. Should nursing and health care education leaders advocate for the inclusion of curricula focusing on grit and resilience?
4. Can health care professionals who lack grit and resilience provide empathetic care in the face of a health crisis?

References

Alexander, C. (2021). *Year of the nurse: A 2020 COVID-19 pandemic memoir.* Caskara Press.

Crow, S., Howard, A.F., Vanderspank-Wright, B., Gillis, P., McLeod, F., Penner, C., & Haljan, G. (2021). The effect of COVID-19 pandemic on the mental health of Canadian critical care nurses providing patient care during the early phase pandemic: A mixed method study. *Journal of Intensive & Critical Care Nursing, 63,* 1–8. https://doi.org/10.1016/j.iccn.2020.102999

Hao, Q., Wang, D., Xie, M., Tang, Y., Dou, Y., Zhu, L., Wu, Y., Dai, M., Wu, H., & Wang, Q. (2021). Prevalence and risk factors of mental health problems among healthcare workers during the COVID-19 pandemic: A systematic review and meta-analysis. *Frontiers in Psychiatry, 12.* https://doi.org/10.3389/fpsyt.2021.567381

Jahner, S., Penz, K., & Stewart, N. J. (2019). Psychological impact of traumatic events in rural nursing practice: An integrative review. *Online Journal of Rural Nursing and Health Care, 19*(1), 105–135. https://doi.org/10.14574/ojrnhc.v19i1.523

Jahner, S., Penz, K., Stewart, N. J., & MacLeod, M. L. P. (2020). Exploring the distressing events and perceptions of support experienced by rural and remote nurses: A thematic analysis of national survey data. *Workplace Health & Safety, 68*(10), 480–490. https://doi.org/10.1177/2165079920924685

Lenthall, S., Wakerman, J., Opie, T., Dollard, M., Dunn, S., Knight, S, MacLeod, M., & Watson, C. (2009). What stresses remote area nurses? Current knowledge and future action. *Australian Journal of Rural Health, 17,* 208–213. http://doi.org/10.1111/j.1440-1584.2009.01073.x

MacLeod, M. L. P., Penz, K. L., Banner, D., Jahner, S., Koren, I. Thomlinson, A., Moffitt, P., & Labrecque, M. E. (2022). Mental health nursing practice in rural and remote Canada: Insights from a national survey. *International Journal of Mental Health Nursing, 31*(1), 128–141. https://doi.org/10.1111/inm.12943

Pappa, S., Sakkas, N., Sakka, E. (2021). A year in review: sleep dysfunction and psychological distress in healthcare workers during COVID-19 pandemic. *Sleep Medicine, 91,* 237–245.

Terry, D., Lê, Q., Nguyen, U., & Hoang, H. (2015). Workplace health and safety issues among community nurses: A study regarding the impact on providing care to rural consumers. *BMJ Open, 5*(8). http://doi.org/10.1136/bmjopen-2015-008306

Trusted Health. (2022). *2022 Frontline nurse mental health & wellbeing survey.* https://assets-global.website-files.com/62991a992ad4fe937e88efec/62d1ba32d9f1be54b8361503_Trusted%20Health%202022%20Mental%20Health%20Survey.pdf

World Health Organization. (2022). *World failing in "our duty of care" to protect mental health and well-being of health and care workers, finds report on impact of COVID-19.* https://www.who.int/news/items/05-10-2022-world

Image Credits

Fig. 8.1: Source: https://mhanational.org/mental-health-healthcare-workers-covid-19.

Fig. 8.2: Source: https://assets-global.website-files.com/62991a992ad4fe937e88efec/62d-1ba32d9f1be54b8361503_Trusted%20Health%202022%20Mental%20Health%20Survey.pdf.

Fig. 8.3: Source: https://assets-global.website-files.com/62991a992ad4fe937e88efec/62d-1ba32d9f1be54b8361503_Trusted%20Health%202022%20Mental%20Health%20Survey.pdf.

Fig. 8.4: Source: https://assets-global.website-files.com/62991a992ad4fe937e88efec/62d-1ba32d9f1be54b8361503_Trusted%20Health%202022%20Mental%20Health%20Survey.pdf.

Fig. 8.5: Source: https://assets-global.website-files.com/62991a992ad4fe937e88efec/62d-1ba32d9f1be54b8361503_Trusted%20Health%202022%20Mental%20Health%20Survey.pdf.

Fig. 8.6: Source: https://assets-global.website-files.com/62991a992ad4fe937e88efec/62d-1ba32d9f1be54b8361503_Trusted%20Health%202022%20Mental%20Health%20Survey.pdf.

CHAPTER 9

Mental Health Care Access During a Time of Crisis

Mental health care in the United States has always been challenging. There are shortages of providers, especially those who have prescriptive capabilities. There are also stigmas and associated treatment from family and friends who have their own mental health challenges. Add these challenges to the crisis of the COVID-19 pandemic and mental health care became even more acute. Approximately one fifth of the U.S. population lives in a rural area, with approximately one fifth of those living in rural areas having some form of mental illness (Morales et al., 2020). However, U.S. adults living in rural areas receive mental health treatment less frequently and from providers with less specialized training than their urban counterparts. Prior to the COVID-19 pandemic, many adults in the United States could not receive mental health care because of health professional shortage areas (Cai et al., 2022) where they resided. It is estimated that 60% of rural residents live in a designated mental health provider shortage area (Morales et al., 2020). Because of this shortage, many rural residents receive their psychiatric care from their primary care provider, but this contributes to the very dismal potential for mental health care for rural residents (Finley, 2020).

Improving Access to Mental Health Care During a Pandemic

The utilization of innovative approaches to mental health care have not been as consistent in rural America, but some progress has been made, especially with the increased use of telehealth. Telehealth has been successful in addressing the lack of mental health providers in rural and remote areas. Telehealth services help to increase access to care in areas with limited mental health resources, provide effective treatment for mental health conditions, and improve medication adherence (Rural Health Information Hub, 2021). There has been an increase in the utilization of telehealth since the start of the pandemic; however, this use is lower in rural areas than in urban areas, with the number of appointments for rural residents 25%–30% lower than appointments in urban areas (Patel, Mehotra et al., 2021; Patel, Rose, & Barnett, 2021). While telehealth visits in rural areas increased from 11 to 147 visits per 1,000 patients, telehealth growth was higher in urban areas, increasing from 7 to 220 visits per 1,000 patients (Chu et al., 2021).

The value of telehealth, especially in the treatment of patients with mental health problems, proved to be a real game-changer. Prior to the pandemic, there was resistance from providers to utilize the telehealth system. Reasons for this included lack of knowledge of the system and capacity, lack of training in the delivery of care via telehealth, and a mistrust of the patient's ability to express satisfaction with telehealth care. Research indicates that reasons for this include (a) misconception about the efficacy or equality of care, (b) believing patients do not prefer this modality, (c) issues with technology, (d) concern over reimbursement or policy, and (e) lack of comfort or education with the overall use of telepsychiatry (Brannen, 2021).

The WHO defines *telehealth* "as the delivery of health care service at a distance using electronic means for 'the diagnosis of treatment, and prevention of disease and injuries, research and evaluation, education of health care providers' to improve well-being (Arafat et al., 2021, para. 2). Telehealth has been used to successfully treat patients with depression, anxiety, and other mental health diagnoses. This was particularly important as the pandemic had a severe psychological impact on rural residents and health care professionals, especially due to isolation and social distancing. Telehealth has been utilized for the past 60 years, and research indicates that clinical outcomes for patients are similar using either telepsychiatry or face-to-face services (Chakrabarti, 2015; Chakrabarti & Shah, 2016; De Las Cuevas et al., 2006; Hubley et al., 2016; O'Reilly et al., 2007).

From 2018 to 2021, there was a significant decline of in-patient visits across the life span (Acharya et al., 2023; Figure 9.1). The decrease of in-patient visits and the utilization of behavioral mental health services had an impact on individuals' lives; as utilization decreased, there was an increase in stress, social isolation, and growing behavioral mental health needs that required greater treatment options. Preliminary data from the CDC (Czeisler et al., 2020), Kaiser Family Foundation (Panchal et al., 2023), and the American Medical Association (AMA; Sarfraz et al., 2021) indicated an increase in the number of adults who reported adverse behavioral health conditions related to the pandemic:

- Forty percent of respondents reported at least one adverse behavioral condition related to the pandemic. They reported symptoms of anxiety, depression, trauma, stress-related disorders, or starting or increasing substance use to cope with stress or emotions (Czeisler et al., 2020).

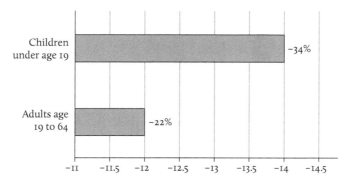

FIGURE 9.1 Decrease in utilization of mental health services (in millions).

- Emergency department visits for overdoses increased 20% in 2019 (Czeisler et al., 2020).
- Suicide attempts from mid-March to mid-October 2020 rose 26% (Czeisler et al., 2020).
- Shelter in-place orders increased rates of suicidal ideation (Czeisler et al., 2020).
- There was a 12% increase in alcohol consumption or substance use to cope with stress and worry (Panchal et al., 2023).
- Every state reported an increase in overdose deaths or substance use disorders during the pandemic (Sarfraz et al., 2021).

The pandemic led to a slowdown in health care service for LGBTQ+ populations, impacting both their physical and behavioral health needs. Sears et al. (2021) noted that during the pandemic LGBTQ adults were more likely to be laid off (12.4% versus 7.8%) or furloughed (14.1% versus 9.7%). This resulted in a decreased ability to pay their mortgage or pay their rent or afford basic household goods compared to non-LGBTQ peers. During the pandemic LGBTQ+ individuals also experienced delays in access to gender-affirming care and diminished social support (Woulfe & Wald, 2020). LQBTQ+ youth experienced higher rates of mental health issues during the pandemic, with 73% from ages 13 to 17 reporting symptoms of anxiety, 67% reporting a depressive disorder, and nearly 50% considering suicide (Woulfe & Wald, 2020).

The pandemic also had an impact on underrepresented populations (Figure 9.2). Individuals from underrepresented populations historically experience higher rates of behavioral mental health conditions and greater barriers to care (AHA, 2022). This includes the following:

- Hispanic adults report higher rates of depression, suicidal ideation, and substance use disorders than Black and White Americans.
- Compared to the general population, Hispanic and Black Americans have gone without behavioral health treatment.
- Black Americans report increase substance use and serious considerations of suicide more frequently than White and Asian counterparts.
- Black and Hispanic adults experienced higher rates of illness and death from COVID-19, negative financial impacts, and poor mental health outcomes.

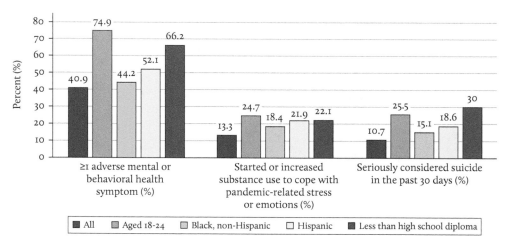

FIGURE 9.2 Prevalence of behavioral health conditions, June 2020.

Within the last 10 years, there has been an increasing number of large-scale, randomized controlled trials that indicate that telepsychiatry is equivalent, or in some cases superior, to face-to-face visits for clinical outcomes (Brannen, 2021). As CMS and private insurance companies assess changes in financial support and reimbursement issues of telehealth, internet and broadband improves for remote parts of the country, and providers become more comfortable in this type of care delivery, those with mental health concerns in rural and remote settings, especially for health care professionals, should realize better and more consistent plans of treatment.

Mental Health Treatment

The need to provide health care providers with the resources, including education for de-escalation and violence intervention, techniques and communication, specialty consultation availability, and other options including organizational and professional support (MacLeod et al., 2022) has potential to reduce mental health challenges for providers. This need is more evident in rural health care settings where there is a shortage of physician providers. In these situations, the trained bedside caregiver may be able to squelch the emergent/urgent situation with the ability to reassure the patient of resources that will help and knowledge of effective communication that the escalated patient find reliable.

The Challenges and Opportunities of Referrals

Care models have demonstrated successful outcomes, including increasing numbers of nonphysician mental health providers such as psychiatric mental health nurse practitioners (PMHNPs). While the parameters of practice are inconsistent from state to state for PMHNPs, there are efforts to decrease regulations and improve reimbursement across state lines for the provision of care to so many in need. Models of care that also support those health care providers HCPs in rural and remote settings include integrative care, medical-assisted treatment (MAT), and value-based care. Integrative care is synonymous with whole-person or patient-centered care and refers to care with consideration of two or more approaches. It involves the optimal combination of evidence-based approaches, including conventional care and drug-free approaches that include complementary and alternative medicine to facilitate healing (Jonas & Rosenbaum, 2021). This model can utilize all types of community members who may not be traditional caregivers in rural and remote settings, resulting in increased resources for those struggling with mental health issues.

Medical-assisted treatment (MAT) is a care model frequently used for substance abuse under the supervision of a provider that uses medications in combination with counseling and behavioral modification therapies for recovery. The providers for this type of treatment are MAT waiver and until 2022 needed to complete courses certified through Substance Abuse and Mental Health Services Administration (SAMHSA, 2023). Laypersons can also serve as support systems for these clients, very similar to the Alcoholics Anonymous (AA) model that incorporates community resources.

Value-based care is a care model that rewards providers with good patient outcomes. Initiated by Centers for Medicare and Medicaid Services (CMS) in 2008, it identifies distinct measures that providers need to meet from performance standards and is tied directly to reimbursement. Areas of psychiatric problems that are covered with value-based care include diagnosis of schizophrenia, depression, alcoholism and drug dependency, and bipolar disorder (Belatti & Lykke, 2018). CMS supports this particular care model as the tangible outcomes established are defined. Providers have the potential to enhance reimbursement for their care if patients can maintain consistent outcomes.

CASE STUDY 9.1

Hospital administration worked hard to support nurses during the pandemic. This support came in the form of staffing, equipment, and sometimes pay increases. Michael, a new chief executive officer (CEO), saw the impact the pandemic had on his staff's mental health, so he implemented some changes. He arranged for on-call counselors to be available at any time for all hospital staff. The hospital is in a very religious community, so Michael understood the need for spiritual support. He established a very strong spiritual care team within the hospital to make sure there was always somebody from spiritual care available to allow not only the families but staff time to talk. He ensured all staff were given contact phone numbers that they could call anonymously. Michael was involved in a media campaign, which was set up for school groups to arrive at the front of the hospital with posters and send letters to support the staff.

He also started making little video chats on a weekly basis to keep staff updated on what was going on with the pandemic, which has continued due to positive feedback. He always ends his video with, "Be kind to yourselves and be kind to others."

Michael noticed the impact his changes made during the pandemic, so he continues to support the staff. He continues the support opportunities, such as weekly luncheon events people can go to if they are available to decompress. He continues to have a positive outlook by posting signs throughout the hospital telling the staff that they just need to get through today and that tomorrow is going to be better to try to build morale.

He elicited nursing administration to be present. Staff stated, "It was nice because they saw nursing administrators that they hadn't seen in a while going around the hospital to check on the nurses, and maybe they brought them a donut or some coffee or some water or whatever, but they were coming around and just being with us, which was nice."

Conclusion

While mental health needs increased during the pandemic, including those of health care professionals, innovative ways to care for these needs have opened doors to address the shortages of opportunities for treatment for those who suffer from psychiatric challenges, including depression, anxiety, drug and alcohol abuse, suicidal thoughts, and other defined mental health diagnoses. Despite the shortages of providers in rural settings, the use of telehealth and of care models that incorporate community resources and nonphysician providers not previously considered have the potential to address mental health care. Access to experts for mental health treatments with consulting groups via telehealth has real potential for addressing the shortage of providers as well as for managing emergent situations.

Questions for Discussion Related to Case Study 9.1

1. What type of support was Michael demonstrating? Please explain the rationale for your choice.
2. What other changes could he have made to support the staff? What obstacles do you anticipate he will face and from whom?

References

Acharya, M., Ali, M. M., Hayes, C. J., Bogulski, C. A., Magann, E. F., & Eswaran, H. (2023). Trends in telehealth visits during pregnancy, 2018 to 2021. *JAMA Network Open*, *6*(4), e236630. https://doi.org/10.1001/jamanetworkopen.2023.6630

American Hospital Association. (May 2022). *TrendWatch: The impacts of the COVID-19 pandemic on behavioral health.* https://www.aha.org/system/files/media/file/2022/05/trendwatch-the-impacts-of-the-covid-19-pandemic-on-behavioral-health.pdf

Arafat, M. Y., Zaman S., & Hawlader, M. D. H. (2021). Telemedicine improves mental health in COVID-19 pandemic. *Journal of Global Health*, *11*. https://doi.org/10.7189/jogh.11.03004

Belatti, D., & Lykke, M. (2018). Diagnosis coding for value-based payment: A quick reference tool. *Family Practice Management*, *25*(2), 26–30. https://www.aafp.org/pubs/fpm/issues/2018/0300/p26.html#:~

Brannen, H. J. (2021). *Evaluating provider opinion of telepsychiatry* [Unpublished doctoral scholarly project]. Montana State University.

Cai, A., Mehrotra, A., Germack, H. D., Busch, A. B., Huskamp, H. A. & Barnett, M. L. (2022). Trends in mental health care delivery by psychiatrists and nurse practitioners in Medicare, 2011–19. *Health Affairs*, *41*(9), 1222–1230. https://doi.org/10.1377/hlthaff.2022.00289

Chakrabarti, S. (2015). Usefulness of telepsychiatry: A critical evaluation of videoconferencing-based approaches. *World Journal of Psychiatry*, *5*(3), 286. https://doi.org/10.5498/wjp.v5.i3.286

Chakrabarti, S., & Shah, R. (2016). Telepsychiatry in the developing world: Whither promised joy? [Review Article]. *Indian Journal of Social Psychiatry*, *32*(3), 273–280. https://doi.org/10.4103/0971-9962.193200

Chu. C., Cram, P., Pang, A., Stamenova, V., Tadrous, M., & Bhatia, R. S. (2021). Rural telemedicine use before and during the COVID-19 pandemic: Repeated cross-sectional study. *Journal of Medical Internet Research*, *23*(4), e26960. https://doi.org/10.2196/26960

Czeisler, M. E., Lane, R. I., Petrosky, E., Wiley, J. F., Christensen, A., Njai, R., Weaver, M. D., Robbins, R., Facer-Childs, E. R., Barger, L. K., Czeisler, C. A., Howard, M. E., & Rajaratnam, S. M. W. (2020). Mental health, substance use, and suicidal ideation during the COVID-19 pandemic–United States, June 24–30, 2020. *Morbidity and Mortality Weekly Report*, *69*(32), 1049–1057. https://www.cdc.gov/mmwr/volumes/69/wr/mm6932a1.htm#:~:text=Overall%2C%2040.9%25%20of%20respondents%20reported,increased%20substance%20use%20to%20copy

De Las Cuevas, C., Arredondo, M. T., Cabrera, M. F., Sulzenbacher, H., & Meise, U. (2006). Randomized clinical trial of telepsychiatry through videoconference versus face-to-face conventional psychiatric treatment. *Telemedicine Journal and E-Health: The Official Journal of the American Telemedicine Association*, *12*(3), 341. https://doi.org/10.1089/tmj.2006.12.341

Hubley, S., Lynch, S. B., Schneck, C., Thomas, M., & Shore, J. (2016). Review of key telepsychiatry outcomes. *World Journal of Psychiatry*, *6*(2), 269–282. https://doi.org/10.5498/wjp.v6.i2.269

Finley, B. A. (2020). Psychiatric mental health nurse practitioners meeting rural mental health challenges. *Journal of the American Psychiatric Nurses Association*, *26*(1). 97–101. https://doi.org/10.1177/1078390319886357

Jonas, W. B., & Rosenbaum, E. (2021). The case for whole-person integrative care. *Medicina*, *57*, 677. https://doi.org/10.3390/medicina57070677

MacLeod, M. L. P., Penz, K. L., Banner, D., Jahner, S., Koren, I. Thomlinson, A., Moffitt, P., & Labrecque, M. E. (2022). Mental health nursing practice in rural and remote Canada: Insights from a national survey. *International Journal of Mental Health Nursing*, *31*(1), 128–141. https://doi.org/10.1111/inm.12943

Morales, D. A., Barksdale, C. L., & Beckel-Mitchener, A. C. (2020). A call to action to address rural mental health disparities. *Journal of Clinical and Translational Science, 4*, 463–467. https://doi.org/10.1017/cts.2020.42

O'Reilly, R., Bishop, J., Maddox, K., Hutchinson, L., Fisman, M., & Takhar, J. (2007). Is telepsychiatry equivalent to face-to-face psychiatry? Results from a randomized controlled equivalence trial. *Psychiatric Services, 58*(6), 836–843. https://doi.org/10.1176/ps.2007.58.6.836

Panchal, N., Saunders, H., Rudowitz, R., & Cox, C. (2023). *The implications of COVID-19 for mental health and substance use.* Kaiser Family Foundation. https://www.kff.org/mental-health/issue-brief/the-implications-of-covid-19-for-mental-health-and-substance-use/

Patel, S. Y., Mehrotra, A., Huskamp, H. A., Uscher-Pines, L., Ganguli, I., & Barnett, M. L. (2021). Variation in telemedicine use and outpatient care during the COVID-19 pandemic in the United States. *Health Affairs, 40*(2), 349–358. https://doi.org/10.1377/hlthaff.2020.01786

Patel, S. Y., Rose, S., & Barnett, M. L. (2021). Community factors associated with telemedicine use during the COVID-19 pandemic. *JAMA Network Open, 4*(5). https://doi.org/10.1001/jamanetworkopen.2021.10330

Rural Health Information Hub. (2022). *Healthcare access in rural communities.* https://www.ruralhealthinfo.org/topics/healthcare-access

Sarfraz, Z., Sarfraz, A., Sarfraz, M., Pandav, K., & Michel, G. (2021). Ripple collision of three epidemics: Vaping, opioid use, and COVID-19. *Addiction & Health, 13*(4), 277–278. https://doi.org/10.22122/ahj.v13i4.303

Substance Abuse and Mental Health Services Administration. (2023). *Waiver elimination (MAT Act).* https://www.samhsa.gov/medications-substance-use-disorders/waiver-elimination-mat-act

Sears, B., Conron, K.J. & Flores, A. R. (2021). *The impact of the fall COVID-19 surge on LGBT adults in the US.* https://williamsinstitute.law.ucla.edu/wp-content/uploads/COVID-LGBT-Fall-Surge-Feb-2021.pdf

Woulfe, J. & Wald, M. (2020, September 22). *The impact of the COVID-19 pandemic on the transgender and non-binary community.* Columbia University. https://www.columbiapsychiatry.org/news/impact-covid-19-pandemic-transgender-and-non-binary-community

Image Credits

Fig. 9.1: Source: https://www.aha.org/system/files/media/file/2022/05/trendwatch-the-impacts-of-the-covid-19-pandemic-on-behavioral-health.pdf.

Fig. 9.2: Source: https://www.aha.org/system/files/media/file/2022/05/trendwatch-the-impacts-of-the-covid-19-pandemic-on-behavioral-health.pdf.

CHAPTER 10

The Pandemic's Impact on School-Aged Children

As schools shut down at the beginning of the coronavirus pandemic and children and adolescents were sequestered at home, questions of the benefits of this isolation also began. Many parents delayed well checks with providers, so as schools started to open and students returned to class, the impact of the pandemic, both physically and mentally, was first observed by the school nurse. The school nurse serves as a frontline provider in many schools, both rural and urban. School nurses play a critical role in the health and wellness of school-aged children, especially because many students do not have access to traditional health care. School nurses are active in disease surveillance, disaster preparedness, wellness and chronic disease prevention interventions, immunizations, mental health screening, and chronic disease education. Furthermore, they provide a safety net for our most vulnerable children. One study by Hoke et al. (2021) reinforced that school nurses need to be involved in the planning of school preparedness in the face of a disaster, its reopening, and the development of policies and programs to mitigate infection transmission.

The pandemic exacerbated preexisting stressors in the U.S. behavioral health services for individuals in special populations. The pandemic caused major disruptions in the daily lives of the young people. Children were forced to transition to online classes, working from home and sometimes alone without the support of their peers. These changes led to an increase in the rates of positive suicide-risk screens among pediatric patients. Like adults, the pandemic impacted access to behavioral health service for children. There was a drop in pediatric mental health visits between March and December 2020, which indicates pediatric patients' needs were not met. Unmet needs lead to an increase in the number of emergency department visits among pediatric patients, frequently requiring inpatient treatment.

The American Academy of Pediatrics (Aubrey, 2020) had concerns about the adverse health consequences of school closures due to COVID-19. Some of the health consequences that led to the recommendation to continue with in-person classes were the impact on education, mental health, child abuse and neglect, and nutrition. However, continuing with in-person classes and returning to school came with the risk of exposing students and family members to

COVID-19. In April 2020, 1.5 billion students worldwide were out of school due to social distancing and lockdown effects to reduce COVID-19 cases (Lee, 2020; Viner, 2022).

Mental Health

An analysis completed by Dorn et al. (2021) showed the impact of COVID-19 and school closures on K–12 student learning. Students, on average, were 5 months behind in mathematics and 4 months in reading. The study also highlighted the preexisting opportunity and achievement gaps across minority students. When examining the impact in mathematics, Black students were 6 months behind their counterparts, and students in low-income schools were 7 months behind (Dorn et al., 2021). The impact of COVID-19 and school closures also affected high school students, with a higher number more likely to drop out of school or not go on to postsecondary education, especially students from families that are low income. The crisis not only impacted education, but it also affected the health and well-being of students, with more than 35% of parents surveyed being very to extremely concerned about their child's mental health (Dorn et al., 2021).

Prior to the pandemic, the CDC reported that one in five children had a mental disorder, with only 20% receiving care from a mental health provider. During the pandemic, children needed continued support for changes in their mental health, increasing over the first 2 years of the pandemic. Children were facing child abuse trauma, loss of family members, and anxiety related to the COVID-19 pandemic (Abramson, 2022).

For many children and adolescents, school closures meant a lack of access to the mental health services they received through their schools. School routines and interaction play an important role in the development of coping mechanisms for students with mental health issues, especially depression. It seemed that when schools shut down and everyone isolated, many of these children and adolescents just locked themselves inside their rooms, resulting in increased isolation.

Children with autism spectrum disorder were also at risk. When these children have a disruption in their daily activities, they can become frustrated and short-tempered. Parents were required to step in and continue their child's care, education, and daily activities. Some children also developed depression, resulting in considerable difficulties adjusting to normal life when school resumed (Lee, 2020).

The most reported consequence of the COVID-19 pandemic is the impact on the mental health of both children and adolescents (Ann & Robert H. Lurie Children's Hospital of Chicago, 2021). One year into the pandemic, a study was completed to understand how parents were monitoring and managing their children's mental health. They polled 1,000 U.S. parents to gain an understanding of how the parents felt the pandemic was affecting their children's mental health, what choices they regretted making, and what they had done to address challenges (Ann & Robert H. Lurie Children's Hospital of Chicago, 2021). Seventy-one percent stated the pandemic had affected their child, 69% stated the pandemic was the worst thing to happen to their child, and 67% stated they wished they had been more observant about their child's mental health. Factors the parents cited for these changes included social isolation, remote learning, amount of screen time, fear of the virus, lack of physical activity, and the news (Figure 10.1).

The pillars of mental health include socialization, which was impacted by school closures and social distancing and exercising, which was impacted by school and local sports activities closures, as well as eating and sleeping. Parents cited social isolation as the unhealthiest aspect of the pandemic, followed by remote learning, which increased screen time (Figure 10.2).

Due to the changes in access to mental health treatment for children, many parents needed to support their child's mental health. Parents reported trying multiple approaches to engage their children (Ann & Robert H. Lurie Children's Hospital of Chicago, 2021):

- talking and comforting their child (63%)
- encouraging their child to pursue hobbies and fun activities (56%)
- encouraging better sleep (42%)
- encouraging more physical activity (40%)
- using mindfulness and relaxation (37%)
- improving diet (33%)
- utilizing virtual socializing (30%)
- increasing in-person socializing (22%)

Child Abuse and Neglect

The U.S. Department of Health and Human Services (2021) estimated that in 2019, there were 7,880,400 referrals for child abuse and neglect (CAN) in the United States, with approximately 3,476,000 screened for a child abuse or neglect investigation (Nguyen, 2021). The COVID-19 pandemic has caused an unprecedented amount of sudden financial, physical, and mental stress. Previous studies have shown that child maltreatment is more likely to occur under these circumstances (Lindo et al., 2018; Lowell & Renk, 2017; Paxson & Waldfogel, 2002). "Social distancing measures can result in social isolation in an abusive home, with abuse likely exacerbated during this time of economic uncertainty and stress" (Lee, 2020, p. 421).

Researchers have examined the impact of disasters, including COVID-19, on child abuse and neglect. Previous research has demonstrated that after natural disasters, there can be an increase in the number of CAN reports (Curtis et al., 2000; Table 10.1).

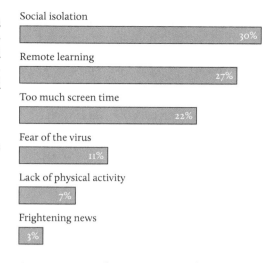

FIGURE 10.1 What parents stated was most unhealthy for their child.

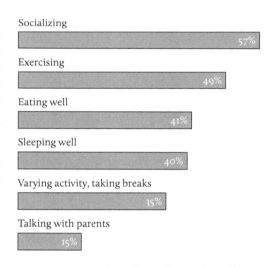

FIGURE 10.2 What pillars of mental health parents stated were compromised during the pandemic.

TABLE 10.1 Impact of Natural Disasters on Child Abuse and Neglect Reports

Event	CAN Reports After 3 Months	CAN Reports After 6 Months	CAN Reports After 1 Year
Hurricane Hugo	Increase of 20.3%	Increase of 19.9%	Increase of 12.5%
Loma Prieta Earthquake	Increase of 9.2%	Increase of 9.0%	Increase of 2.8%
Hurricane Andrew	Decrease of 18%	Decrease of 18.9%	Decrease of 11%

COVID-19 had a major impact on CAN, leading to changes in the number of reported investigations, missed prevention cases, and missed CAN cases (Nguyen, 2021). Secondary analysis of administrative data for New York City, Florida, New Jersey, and Wisconsin from March 2020 to December 2020 was used to determine the number of CAN cases. The 7-year monthly average of CAN investigations for March 2013 through December 2019 was calculated and compared to the numbers of CAN investigations for March 2020 to December 2020 (Nguyen, 2021; Table 10.2).

TABLE 10.2 Number of CAN Investigations from January 2013 to December 2020

Location	7-Year Average	2020	Change From 7-year Average to 2000
New York City	56,541	41, 963	−35.5%
Florida	207,846	171,246	−25.2%
New Jersey	16,812	10,920	−55%
Wisconsin	27,540	27,304	−24%

Teachers and school personnel are some of the largest groups to report child abuse (Baron et al., 2020). Researchers found that all types of child abuse become more frequent during school holidays, summer breaks, and natural disasters (Caron et al., 2020). In addition, women in abusive relationships and their children are at increased risk for domestic violence and abuse when family members spend more time in close contact and when families must cope with additional stress, financial problems, and/or unemployment (Caron et al., 2020). During the pandemic when schools were closed, there were no teachers, school personnel, or nurses monitoring children at risk for abuse. There was "a broken link between reporters and victims of child maltreatment" (Baron et al., 2020, p. 1). Teachers, guidance counselors, school psychologists, and other school workers are mandated reporters of suspected child maltreatment in every state. This group submitted more than any other professional group, with over 20% of the 4.3 million nationwide reports in 2018 (Baron et al., 2020). To understand the impact of school closures on child maltreatment reporting, Baron et al. (2020) collected monthly county-level data on the number of child maltreatment allegations made to the Florida Child Abuse Hotline. They estimated in March and April 2020 that child maltreatment related to COVID-19 led to increases in child maltreatment. However, their findings indicated that approximately 15,000 fewer allegations were reported in March and April 2020 (Baron et al., 2020).

Nutrition

During the first few weeks of the pandemic, more than half of U.S. schools announced closures coinciding with the COVID-19 emergency declarations. These school closures not only impacted the mental health of children but also disrupted access to food. At least 124,000 U.S. public and private schools were impacted, affecting at least 55.1 million students (McLoughlin et al., 2020). This took away a critical nutritional source for more than 30 million children who participated in the U.S. Department of Agriculture's (USDA) National

School Lunch Program (NSLP) and 15 million students who participated in the School Breakfast Program (SBP; McLoughlin et al., 2020). These programs have had a large impact on child food insecurity, but with the closures many students were not able to receive free or reduced school meals (Table 10.3).

TABLE 10.3 Weekly and Cumulative Missed Free and Reduced-Price School Meals, Including Breakfast and Lunch, From March 2 to May 1, 2020

Dates	Weekly Meals	Cumulative
March 2–6	36,802	36,802
March 9–13	2,598,526	2,635,328
March 16–20	124,824,223	127,459,551
March 23–27	169,479,514	296,939,064
March 30–April 3	169,619,512	466,558,576
April 6–10	169,619,512	636,178,088
April 13–17	169,619,512	805,797,601
April 20–24	169,619,512	975,417,113
April 27–May 1	169,619,512	1,145,036,625

Source: Kinsey et al. (2020).

CASE STUDY 10.1

Joshua lives with his single mother and older sister (14 years) in rural Iowa. After school Joshua and his sister go home to an empty house until their mother returns from work. While Joshua's mother knows this is not ideal, she has no choice as she needs to work to maintain the family. However, she still struggles to put food on the table. She is grateful her children receive both breakfast and lunch at school along with food for the weekend. But when the pandemic hit and the schools in their area closed, she was challenged with who was going to watch her children all day and how she was going to feed her children breakfast and lunch. She could not leave her job; if she did not work, she would put her family at risk of losing their home.

In March 2020, to mitigate the number of students who were at risk for food insecurity, Congress granted the USDA flexibilities in how school-based nutrition assistance programs were delivered. This change was important as COVID-19 impacted many Americans' financial status, especially individuals from racial/ethnic minorities, posing further barriers to those who were already food insecure. During the pandemic, it was estimated that food insecurity doubled for individuals with food insecurity and tripled in populations with children. The flexibility granted included increasing school-year reimbursement rates to the level offered during the summer and not requiring that meals be served as a group setting, opening the possibility that food could be prepared and packaged to be picked up by the students or parents. In some areas, meals were delivered using school buses to different neighborhoods throughout the school district (Aubrey, 2022).

Through the challenges of the pandemic and how to offer meals to all school-aged children came innovation (Kinsey et al., 2020). In response to school closures, there was a need to determine how to distribute meals to the students. New distribution sites, mobile distribution using school buses, home delivery in rural areas, and coordination with community partners were initiated. As a result of increased community need, some districts expanded their meal service to 7 days per week, while others offered 1 week of meals at one time to decrease staff exposure and to improve convenience for parents and students. Due to supply chain challenges and staff shortages, some school districts tried to increase meal participation and decrease waste by having students preorder meals online or by phone, allowing them to choose meals that were appealing to them. Many districts also saw the need to expand meal services beyond school-aged children, making meals available to all children 0 to 18 years old and students with disabilities 18 to 26 years old.

Despite these increases in food insecurity and heroic efforts by school food service, the number of students who participated in free meals remained low, and schools were suffering financial losses (McLoughlin et al., 2020). In the 2020–2021 school year, participation in emergency school meals was low, indicating that many students were at increased risk for food insecurity. Due to low enrollment, school meal programs were also at risk of losing federal funding, resulting in all students at risk for food insecurity. As we have emerged from the pandemic, feeding our children continues to be a challenge. The Food Research & Action Center's (FRAC) "Large School District Report" surveyed 62 large school districts in the United States related to the challenges they experienced in providing school meals (Baker, 2022). Of the districts surveyed, 98% identified supply chain disruptions as a challenge, and 95% stated labor shortages were a problem. Despite these challenges, respondents offered school meals to all students at no charge, which had a large impact on the children, their families, and the school district (Baker, 2022). Their findings included the following:

- Ninety-five percent reported the nationwide waivers reduced child hunger in their district.
- Eighty-nine percent reported the waivers made it easier for parents and guardians.
- Eighty-five percent reported that by making meals available to all students at no cost it eliminated the stigma associated with school meals.
- Eighty-four percent reported the nationwide waivers eased administrative work.
- Eighty-two percent reported the nationwide waivers supported academic achievement.

Conclusion

One of the lessons learned from the pandemic was the lack of nutritional food for school age children and their families with the lack of access to school breakfast and lunch programs. "School breakfast and lunch are proven tools for fueling children's health and learning" (Baker, 2022, para 4). Without nutrition and the interaction students receive at school, they are at risk for multiple health, mental health, and social disadvantages.

Questions for Discussion Related to Case Study 10.1

1. What changes did rural school districts make to address food insecurity for the students in their districts when schools were mandated to close?

2. What options did Joshua's mother have to ensure her children were safe during the day when she was at work?
3. How could Joshua's mother ensure her children can continue with their studies, especially when they need internet access, which she cannot afford?

References

Abramson, A. (2022). Children's mental health is in crisis. *Monitor on Psychology*, *53*(1). https://www.apa.org/monitor/2022/01/special-childrens-mental-health

Ann & Robert H. Lurie Children's Hospital of Chicago. (2021). Children's mental health during the COVID-19 pandemic. *Lurie Children's Blog*. https://www.luriechildrens.org/en/blog/childrens-mental-health-pandemic-statistics/

Aubrey, A. (2022, March 21). *Millions of children will miss healthy school meals when pandemic relief expires*. NPR. https://www.npr.org/sections/health-shots/2022/03/21/1087658783/millions-of-children-will-miss-healthy-school-meals-when-pandemic-relief-expires

Baker, J. (2022). *Pandemic child nutrition waivers a game-changer for students, families, schools, report finds*. Food Research & Action Center. https://frac.org/news/largedistrict2022

Baron, E. J., Goldstein, E. G., & Wallace, C. T. (2020). Suffering in silence: How COVID-19 school closures inhibit the reporting of child maltreatment. *Journal of Public Economics*, *190*. https://doi.org/10.1016/j.jpubeco.2020.104258

Caron, F., Plancq, M. C, Tourneuz, P., Gouron, R., & Klein, C. (2020). Was child abuse under-detected during the COVID-19 lockdown? *Archives de Pediatrie*, *27*, 399–401.

Curtis, T., Miller, B. C., & Berry, E. H. (2000). Changes in reports and incidence of child abuse following natural disasters. *Child Abuse & Neglect*, *24*(9), 1151–1162. https://doi.org/10.1016/S0145-2134(00)00176-9

Dorn, E., Hancock, B., Sarakatsannis, J., & Viruleg, E. (2021). *US states and districts have the opportunity to not only help students catch up on unfinished learning from the pandemic but also tackle long-standing historical inequities in education*. McKinsey & Company. https://www. https://www.mckinsey.com/industries/education/our-insights/covid-19-and-education-the-lingering-effects-of-unfinished-learning

Hoke, A. M., Keller, C. M., Calo, W. A., Sekhar, D. L., Lehman, E.B., & Kraschnewski, J. L. (2021). School nurse perspectives on COVID-19. *The Journal of School Nursing*, *37*(4), 292–297.

Kinsey, E. W., Hecht, A. A., Dunn, C. G., Levi, R., Read, M. A., Smith, C., Niesen, P., Seligman, H. K., & Hager, E. R. (2020). School closures during COVID-19: Opportunities for innovation in meal service. *American Journal of Public Health*, *110*(11), 1635–1643.

Lindo, J. M., Schaller, J., & Hansen, B. (2018). Caution! Men not at work: Gender-specific labor market conditions and child maltreatment. *Journal of Public Economics*, *163*, 77–98.

Lee, J. (2020). Mental health effects of school closures during COVID-19. *The Lancet: Child & Adolescent Health*, *4*, 421. https://doi.org/10.1016/S2352-4642(20)30109-7

Lowell, A., & Renk, K. (2017). Predictors of child maltreatment potential in a national sample of mothers of young children. *Journal of Aggression, Maltreatment & Trauma*, *26*, 335–353.

McLoughlin, G. M., Fleischhacker, S., Hecht, A. A., McGuirt, J., Vega, C., Read, M., Colón-Ramos, U., & Dunn, C. G. (2020). Feeding students during COVID-19 related school closures: A nationwide assessment of initial responses. *Journal of Nutrition Education and Behavior*, *52*(12), 1120–1130. https://doi.org/10.1016/j.jneb.2020.09.018

Nguyen, L. H. (2021). Calculating the impact of COVID-19 pandemic on child abuse and neglect in the U.S. *Child Abuse & Neglect*, *118*, 1–12.

Paxson, C., & Waldfogel, J. (2002). Work, welfare, and child maltreatment. *Journal of Labor Economics, 20*, 435–474.

Viner, R., Russell S., Saulle, R., Croker, H., Stansfield, C., Packer, J., Nicholls, D., Goddings, A. Bonell, C., Hudson, L., Hope, S., Ward, J., Schwalbe, N., Morgan, A., & Minozzi, S. (2022). School closures during social lockdown and mental health, health behaviors, and well-being among children and adolescents during the first COVID-19 wave: A systematic review. *JAMA Pediatrics, 176*(4), 400–409. https://doi.org/10.1001/jamapediatrics.2021.5840

Image Credits

Finding Synergy in the Design, Delivery, and Evaluation of Nursing Curriculum

I n early 2020, nursing programs had to abruptly shutter their doors and regroup to a largely remote or online educational model due to the governmental restrictions and student safety issues imposed by the COVID-19 pandemic. Digital technology became the solution for many urban programs that could not offer in-person learning. However, for undergraduate and graduate nursing programs based in rural areas, connectivity and virtual communication is often limited due to geographic and technological barriers. During the COVID-19, simulation and virtual technologies were utilized to help off-set the restrictions that existed in clinical settings. However, these strategies did not or could not replace learning in an on-ground clinical setting.

CHAPTER 11

Supporting Learners Through the Unprecedented

Characteristics that are valued within the nursing profession include empathy, honesty and caring. These characteristics are often developed in clinical settings, where students have an opportunity to interact with instructors, mentors, other health care professionals, and patients. Badowski et al. (2021) conducted a qualitative study on a diverse population of nurses, nurse educators, and nursing students. The study sought to identify the consequences of the pandemic on nursing education and recommendations for change in a post-COVID-19 world. The results highlighted four key themes: teamwork and communication, flexibility and critical thinking, leadership, and finding your voice in the areas of policy and advocacy. The researchers emphasized that interruptions in classroom and clinical learning impeded students from developing both competencies and confidence to meet the needs of persons who are both acutely and chronically ill. One participant noted the challenges of teaching the concept of empathy in a solely virtual world: "You can teach all the knowledge that you can, but you can't teach caring or empathy. ... Nurses must understand the importance of empathy" (p. 4).

In 2020, nursing education experienced a dramatic change in the delivery of didactic and clinical learning experiences. Face-to-face classrooms were shuttered, and students and faculty were forced to switch to online learning modalities quickly. This new reality highlighted the lack of emergency education preparedness that existed across U.S. nursing faculty and university leaders, showing the need to develop a rich, mobile curriculum for students that would address student well-being, adaptation to online learning, and the unique challenges of securing in-person clinical placement experiences.

Meeting Regulatory Requirements

In the United States, the foundation for nursing education consists of a blend of classroom (didactic) and direct patient care (in-person clinical experiences; American Association of Colleges of Nursing [AACN], 2008). Nationally, nursing regulatory bodies, such as AACN and state boards of nursing (National Council of State Boards of Nursing [NCSBN], 2024) set written standards and guidelines on the type and amount of didactic and clinical experiences that students must demonstrate competence in to successfully graduate from a nursing program (NCSBN, 2024). The governmental and public health restrictions enforced during the height of the COVID-19 pandemic threatened nursing students' ability to complete their nursing education on time (Michel et al., 2021).

Perceptions of Undergraduate Nursing Students on Nursing Education

In 2020, a group of nursing researchers from five U.S. universities were encouraged to participate in an online survey to extract both quantitative and qualitative data to better understand the perceptions of undergraduate nursing students on nursing education during the height of the COVID-19 pandemic (Michel et al., 2021). This primary study examined U.S. nursing students' perceptions of how the pandemic influenced their desire to become a nurse and enter the workforce during this public health crisis. The final sample included quantitative data from 772 participants and qualitative data from 540 students. The Perceived Stress Scale (Cohen, 1983) was utilized for this study following an adaptation of the scale using back-translation techniques for the language adaptation of the scale. Data analysis from the study overwhelmingly revealed that the students' experiences during the pandemic increased their desire to become a nurse (65.1%). A small percentage of the students (11%) had considered withdrawing from their nursing programs during the 2020 academic year due to frustration with the lack of clinical experiences and/or family/financial stressors (Michel et al., 2021). Only 1% (five students) indicated they no longer wanted a career in nursing. The qualitative responses from students highlighted the impact of the pandemic on their psychological well-being; the challenges and opportunities of shifting to online learning; and the collaborations they witnessed between their universities and clinical partners. Further analysis of the qualitative data highlighted obstacles to learning that the participants experienced: the lack of communication from the faculty and various universities' administration, increased workloads due to changes in curriculum delivery and content, social and academic isolation, challenges (e.g., time, location, resources) related to learning, and multiple logistics issues (e.g., lack of internet connectivity, limited access to computers, and the necessary software programs to complete their assignments). Although many students reported difficulties in connecting with classmates and instructors during the height of the COVID-19 pandemic using web-based applications, one student detailed that they specifically relied on the internet to connect with other students virtually and how that "expanded [his] collaboration skills" (Michel et al., 2021, p. 906).

An added stressor reported in the findings related to continual changes in school schedules and schools' clinical guidelines. One participant reported, "There is so much uncertainty. ... I am worried that any day my program will go 100% online, or we could be barred from participating in clinical experiences due to rising COVID-19 cases. These concerns have added tremendous stress for me and impacted my ability to learn" (Michel et al., 2021, p. 906). On a positive note, many students reported that communication to students from their school administrators helped them to navigate their learning and alleviate some anxieties. Table 11.1 highlights three themes that emerged from the qualitative data analysis. These results were consistent across all U.S. regions.

The researchers note that these findings are congruent with national and international reports, confirming similar learning obstacles (Aslan & Pekince, 2020; Bawa, 2020;

TABLE 11.1 Qualitative Analysis and Emerging Themes

Themes	Student Responses to Open-Ended Questions
Effect of the pandemic on students' psychosocial well-being	"Not being able to meet freely with other students has been the worst effect of the pandemic" (p. 906). "I feel isolated, and the loss of my study group has made school more difficult" (p. 906).
Students' difficult adjustment to online learning during the pandemic	"I do not learn well in an online school environment, and that is why I didn't sign up for one" (p. 906).
	"It is difficult to stay engaged with the course content and find the motivation to study and complete assignments" (p. 906).
Challenges to obtaining clinical experience and developing nursing skills	"I am a student that needs to use my hands to learn, so remote labs have been a challenge for me" (p. 907).
	"Losing in-person clinical time and learning health assessment in a complete virtual setting has made me feel incredibly underprepared when it comes to my basic nursing skills" (p. 907).

Source: Michel et al. (2021).

Huang et al., 2020). Additionally, these findings are similar to findings among medical and pharmacy students; study participants were concerned about the lack of in-person clinical experiences that they deemed essential to successfully enter the workforce (Baczek et al., 2020; Farooq et al., 2020; Shawaqfef et al., 2020). The researchers point out that these realities highlight a weakness in the nursing education process within the United States, along with schools of nursing educational emergency preparedness, as evidenced by the somewhat frantic transition to emergency remote teaching and the halt of students' abilities to participate in in-person clinical learning experiences (Michel et al., 2021). The Federal Emergency Management Agency (FEMA, 2013) stated that nursing programs must develop comprehensive plans of action for future temporary and/or emergency shifts to online learning. These plans must include addressing the effects of a future disaster on nursing students, clinical site placements, collaborative agreements, and regulatory requirements associated with nursing education.

CASE STUDY 11.1

Olivia is a nursing student at a small rural college studying to become a nurse. Olivia lives about 30 miles from the college but really enjoys driving to the college with one of her friends from the same community. Both she and her friend Jessica come from families with low income, which limits their resources. When the pandemic hit, Olivia and Jessica were preparing to begin their first clinical rotation at the same hospital approximately 40 miles from their community. Unfortunately, due to the pandemic they were told they could not complete their scheduled clinical and that they would be completing their studies via the internet with weekly simulation on campus. Olivia and Jessica did not have access to the internet from their homes; however, they were able to access the internet and thus their classes from the parking lot of the local fire department.

A Preventative Approach: The Early Prevention Methods in Turkey

The COVID-19 pandemic began later in Turkey than in other countries in the European region; however, unlike many other countries, Turkey implemented early intervention protocols to minimize the spread of the virus. These interventions included social distancing, home isolation, the closure of universities and schools, canceling or postponing events and congresses, and travel restrictions (WHO, 2020). However, the abrupt halting of familiar nursing education practices was unexpected by both faculty and students, adding to the uncertainty and stressors experienced by nursing students.

Aslan and Pekince (2021), conducted a study focusing on nursing students attending three universities in Eastern Turkey. The aim of the cross-sectional study was to evaluate nursing students' views and experiences regarding the COVID-19 pandemic and their perceived stress levels. Data were collected utilizing an information form developed by the researchers and the Perceived Stress Scale (PSS). The study participants ranged in age from 18–20 years, with an average age of 20.67 + −1.61 years. More than one half of the students (51.7%) were in the 18–20 age range, 71.9% were female, and 44.4% were in the first year of their nursing program. Study results indicated that 48% of the students often assimilated news about the COVID-19 pandemic, and 91.5% routinely followed news about the virus from other countries (Aslan & Pekince, 2021).

Data analysis revealed that students perceived moderate levels of stress, yet higher levels of stress than students assessed in previous years (Aslan & Pekince, 2021). Table 11.2 compares the demographic variables and the Perceived Stress Scale score of averages. This is significant information for faculty who teach those students who enter nursing programs immediately following high school graduation. Aslan and Pekince (2021) state, "It is thought that the ability to cope with the stress of younger students is not fully developed,

TABLE 11.2 Comparison of Demographic Variables and Perceived Stress Scale Score Averages

| | | Perceived Stress Scale | |
		X + −SD	Test and Significance
Age	18–20	32.94 + −7.10	$t = 1.583$
	21 and above	29.71 + −6.71	$p = .000$
Sex	Female	32.92 +−7.04	$t = 3.793$
	Male	29.57 +−6.71	$p = .000$
Class	1	32.67 + −6.70	$KW = 3.655$
	2	30.59 + −7.08	$p = .301$
	3	30.52 + −6.83	
	4	30.90 + −6.71	
Perceived Stress Scale Total Score	X + −SD		
	31.69 + −6.91		

Key: KW, Kruskal-Wallis Test; SD, standard deviation; t, independent sample t-test; X, mean.

Source: Aslan and Pekince (2021).

and inadequate training received in universities about infectious diseases may have also increased their perceived level of stress" (p. 698). Currently, there is a gap in the literature regarding the age of students, their levels of perceived stress, and the necessary strategies that nursing faculty and universities must have in place to provide students with coping support during a prolonged emergency.

The average score of the PSS was 31.69 + −6.91. Aslan and Pekince (2021) stated that these nursing students experienced moderate stress. It is important to note that significant differences in PSS scores were found in terms of age and sex ($p < .001$ and $p < .001$, respectively). The perceived stress level for students under the age of 20 was significantly higher than those experienced by students aged 20 years or older. The researchers postulate that the curfew that was imposed on students under the age of 20 affected these findings. Aslan and Pekince (2021) suggest that the curfew and the resulting decrease in social activities, limitations on physical activities in the home, and changes in dietary and sleep habits may have influenced the increased stress experienced by these students. "It is thought that the ability to cope with the stress of younger students is not fully developed, and the lack of training provided in university settings at that point in their education may also have increased their level of stress" (Aslan & Pekince, 2021, p. 699). The researchers emphasize the need for universities to infuse the development of skills in nursing students to cope with moderate stress in order to protect themselves, their family members, and the community in their curricula related to epidemic infections.

Conclusion

Findings from research indicate that despite the challenges of the COVID-19 pandemic, students' desire to pursue a career in nursing had strengthened (Michel et al., 2021). However, the events surrounding the pandemic and the crisis surrounding the transition to remote learning negatively impacted students' sense of well-being, created barriers to learning, and highlighted the need for faculty to develop alternative strategies for students to master psychomotor skills and confidence in nursing care to enter practice. There is an emergent need for universities to offer a variety of programs, both virtually and on the ground, for students to socialize and formulate networks for studying and sharing the opportunities and challenges that nursing students encounter throughout their learning experiences. Additionally, there is a need for faculty and university leadership to collaborate on initiatives to meet the needs of students, faculty, and regulatory agencies' mandates for graduation and licensure. Therefore, research examining the effectiveness of online learning simulation and novel strategies for providing clinical experiences must continue. Ongoing collaborations and alliances between nursing programs and health care organizations will help ensure that the United States produces adequately trained nurses who can provide safe patient care to address the growing staffing crisis.

Questions for Discussion Related to Case Study 11.1

1. What changes could have been made to ensure Olivia and Jessica could attend their hospital clinical as scheduled?
2. What was the impact of limited internet access for students needing to study from their homes and rural communities?
3. What was the impact of the changes made in nursing education to the preparation of nurses? What support will they need in their first job to be successful?

References

American Association of Colleges of Nursing. (2008). *The essence of baccalaureate education for professional nursing practice.* https://www.aacnnursing.org/portals/42/publications/baccessentials08.pdf.

Aslan, H., & Pekince, H. (2021). Nursing students' views on the COVID-19 pandemic and their perceived stress levels. *Perspectives in Psychiatric Care, 57*(2), 695–701. https://doi.org/10.1111/ppc.12597

Badowski, D. M., Spurlark, R., Webber-Ritchey, K. J., Towson, S., Ponder, T. N., & Simonvich, S.D. (2021). Envisioning nursing education for a post? COVID-19 world: Qualitative findings from the frontline. *Journal of Nursing Education, 60*(1), 1–10. http://doi.org/10.3928/01484834-20211004-03

Baczek, M., Zagancyk-Baczek, M., Szpinger, M., Jaroszynski, A., & Wozakowska-Kaplon, B. (2020). Students' perception of online learning during the COVID-19 pandemic: A survey study of Polish medical students. *Medicine, 100*(7), 1–6. https://doi.org/10.1016/MD.0000000000024821

Bawa, P. (2020). Learning in the age of SARS-COV-2: A quantitative study of learners' performance in the age of emergency remote teaching. *Computers and Education Open, 1.* https://doi.org/.10.1016/j.caeo.2020.100016

Cohen, S., Kamarck, T., & Mermelstein, R. (1983). A Global Measure of Perceived Stress. *Journal of Health and Social Behavior, 24*(4), 385-396, Retrieved from https://doi.org/10.2307/2136404

Farooq, F., Rathore, F., & Mansoor, S. (2020). Challenges of online medical education in Pakistan during COVID-19 pandemic. *Journal of the College of Physicians and Surgeons Pakistan, 30*(6), 67–69. https://doi.org/10.29271/jcpsp.2020.Suppl.S67

Federal Emergency Management Agency. (2013). *Guide for developing high quality emergency operations plans for institutions of higher learning.* https://www.ready.gov/sites/default/files/2020-03/emergency-operations-plans_institution-higher-education.pdf

Huang, L., Lei, W., Xu, F., Liu, H., & Yu, L. (2020). Emotional responses and coping strategies in nurses and nursing students during Covid-19 outbreak: A comparative study. *PLoS, 15*(8), e0237303. https://doi.org/10.1371/journal.pone.0237303

Michel, A., Ryan, N., Mattheus, D., Knopf, A., Abuelezam, N. N., Stamp, K., Branson, S., Hekel, B., & Fontenot, H. B. (2021). Undergraduate nursing students' perceptions on nursing education during the 2020 COVID-19 pandemic: A national sample. *Nursing Outlook, 69*(5), 903–912. https://doi.org/10.1016/j.outlook.2021.05.004

National Council of State Boards of Nursing. (2024). *Board of nursing licensure requirements.* https://www.ncsbn.org/nursing-regulation/education/board-of-nursing-licensure-requirements.page

Shawaqfeh, M., Al Bekairy, A., Al-Azayzih, A., Alkatheri, A., Qandil, A., Obaidat, A., Harbi, S., & Muflih, S (2020). Pharmacy students perceptions of their distance online learning experience during the COVID-19 pandemic: A cross-sectional survey study. *Journal of Medical Education and Curricular Development, 7,* 1–9. https://doi.org/10.1177/ 2382120520963039

World Health Organization. (2020). *Getting your workplace ready for COVID-19.* https://www.who.int/docs/default-source/coronaviruse/getting-workplace-ready-for-covid-19.pdf

CHAPTER 12

Preserving a Sense of Belonging Amidst Illness and Immunizations

Nurses often receive encouragement and support from their peers. However, the disruptions that were a result of the COVID-19 pandemic set up many for a lack of this support. Increase of burnout, fear of virus exposure and their own health and safety, vaccine hesitancy, and inconsistent practice standards all contributed to insecurity and a lack of a sense of belonging, especially evident in rural and remote settings. In 2020, Dos Santos began to examine the desire and reasons that influenced the experiences, sense of belonging, and career trajectory decisions of nursing students in Japan. The researcher interviewed participants both prior to the COVID-19 pandemic and during the pandemic. The results of the interviews highlighted the commitment that Japanese nursing students felt for the strength of Japan's health care workforce. That commitment superseded their own personal development and goals: "Many people in the housing facilities need regular assistance from nurses. ... I felt so bad because we missed some visits during the height of COVID-19 pandemic ... as nursing students, many of my classmates joined volunteer services so that we could continue to help" (Dos Santos, 2020, p. 10). Although many of the participants had an opportunity to drop their nursing majors during this time, few students left their nursing programs. They felt it was their mission to serve their country (Dos Santos, 2020).

In 2017, the U.S. Department of Health and Human Services, Health Resources and Service Administration (HRSA, 2017) documented the projected demand for registered nurses to increase from 2.8 million in 2014 to 3.6 million by 2030. According to Walker et al. (2018), this projection was based on health care needs and staffing patterns throughout urban and rural areas and the retirement of baby boomer nurses due to dissatisfaction in the workplace. However, these projections were made prior to the onset of the COVID-19 pandemic. Sablik (2022) describes these barriers as emergent public health problems, particularly in rural areas. In a February 2021 interview, Michael Topchik, a national leader for Chartis Center for Rural Health, stated, "When a hospital closes because of staffing concerns, you are talking about Suzie sliding into third base and not being able to get the comfort of care when she breaks her ankle" (Ross, 2021, para. 2).

In November 2021, the Chartis Group, a health care advisory organization, reported that they viewed the nursing shortage as a barrier to providing care in rural hospitals. Sablik (2022) stated that 27% of 130 rural hospital leaders reported having to turn away patients and halt some patient care services completely due to the nursing shortage (Figure 12.1). Wakefield et al. (2023) stated that the ongoing physical and psycho-social demands of responding to the needs of patients with COVID-19 and their families have increased job-related stress for nurses. In some settings, normalized practices such as mandated overtime to cover staffing shortages are increasingly reported.

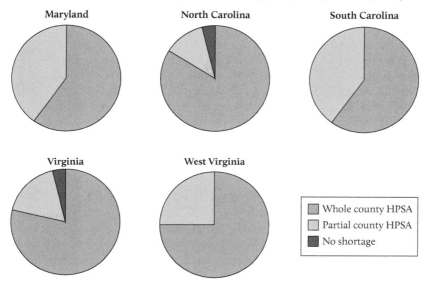

Most Rural Counties in the Fifth District Face Health Workforce Shortages
Share of nonmetro counties with health professional shortages for primary care as of January 2022

NOTE: "HPSA" stands for Health Professional Shortage Area, as designated by the Health Resources and Services Administration.

FIGURE 12.1 Rural counties in HRSA's fifth U.S. district facing workforce shortages.

Nurse Burnout

Mudallal et al. (2017) describe nurse burnout as a prevalent phenomenon defined by decreases in nurses' energy that manifests in emotional fatigue, decreased motivation, and feelings of hopelessness, which may lead to reduced work efficacy. There has been a gap in the literature about the nursing workforce nationally and internationally over the last decade, and staffing shortages continue to worsen as the nursing workforce ages. Willis et al. (2016) described rural hospital nursing as a professional isolating phenomenon, lacking the support of management and with narrowed pathways to continuing education and career advancement. Sellers et al. (2019) expanded on rural nurses' barriers, including limited housing options and inadequate services available for nurses interested in relocating to rural settings. These barriers were further exacerbated when the COVID-19 virus spread and governmental shutdowns further impacted local communities.

Smith et al. (2019) examined rural nurses' barriers in Australia and the relationship between job satisfaction, stress, and nursing burnout. Findings from the research indicated that nurses working in small rural hospitals have high levels of job satisfaction; as nurse managers demonstrated job satisfaction as a value for their nursing staff, there was a higher retention rate among nurses and improved patient safety and quality of care.

This study highlighted that effective, interdisciplinary communication, staffing and resource capabilities, nurse manager skills and leadership abilities, mentoring and role modeling for nurses, compassion fatigue, and intention to leave nursing within 5 years were predictors of nurse burnout and retention (Smith et al., 2019). The demands placed on nurses during the COVID-19 pandemic worsened each of these factors. Nursing leaders must take a broader view to preserve and strengthen the current workforce in rural settings to prioritize patient safety and minimize nurse burnout.

Short et al. (2019) state that newly graduated registered nurses comprise 42% of the annual new-hire workforce. However, many new nurses leave the profession due to a lack of professional belonging and support (Wakefield et al., 2022). Levett-Jones and Lathlean (2008) describe newly licensed registered nurses' desire for acceptance, belonging, care, and encouragement from their colleagues. Strategies designed to achieve this feeling of belonging center around a "healthy" workplace environment with adequate mentoring support and an emphasis on belonging. Mentoring and support have been linked to reducing transition shock for new registered nurses and enhanced feelings of belonging. The concept of rural culture and support for that culture in health care was researched by Sharp (2010) when she studied the impact of rural culture on nurse practitioners and their care of rural dwellers. Sharp wrote that she achieved honesty, meaning, and credibility because of the time she spent establishing trust with rural residents as an APRN in a rural community. Her clinical practice experience allowed her to gain an understanding of both rural culture and the challenges that were common for advanced practice registered nurses (APRNs) to face daily when caring for members of rural communities. Researchers and care providers who have a rural background and understand both the unique attributes of the culture and health care needs of rural and remote communities may be able to gain access and establish trust with residents in these communities more easily (Farmer et al., 2012).

Knighten (2022) stated that there is an abundance of evidence that formal orientation programs can decrease turnover, bridge the transition to practice gap, and support the transition of new graduates into professional nursing practice. The researcher identifies two well-known programs, Versant and Vizient, that provide 1-year residency transition to practice programs (Knighten, 2022).

The Versant program is based on a competency-based model that focuses on each nurse within a specialty, highlights areas of need using a gap analysis, and remediates those needs before validation occurs at the point of care. Debriefing and mentoring a foundational construct within the model have resulted in improvements in retention. The company reports turnover rates of 4.9% in the 1st year and 14% at 24 months (Goode et al., 2018). These rates are significantly lower than the national turnover rates, which estimate that 18% new nurses exit their roles within their 1st year after graduation and 33.3% of new nurses leave within the first 2 years (Lockhart, 2020).

In 1999, the Versant New Graduate RN Residency (NRP) accepted its first applicants at Children's Hospital Los Angeles. The program began as a research project that aimed to determine whether a formalized NRP could increase new graduate nurse competency, confidence, satisfaction, and retention (Ulrich et al., 2010). The Versant NRP uses Benner's novice-to-expert framework as its foundation. The program includes a curriculum with classroom content, clinical experiences focusing on patients with multisystem needs and supported by a trained preceptor, formal mentoring sessions, and debriefing and unique self-care programs. New nurses are paired with other new nurses who have similar levels of experience. As the program progresses, the new nurses are assigned to individual nurses who are experts in their nursing specialty. The program is open to nurses with various educational backgrounds, including diploma graduates through master's-level nurses.

Vizient and the American Association of Colleges of Nursing (AACN) jointly developed a residency program more than 20 years ago. The program requires an academic-practice partnership between the hospital and a nursing school as a condition of participation. Vizient's model includes clinical experiences guided by experienced mentors, participation in monthly didactic seminars, and small group activities. The program's retention rate is reported at 93% at the 1-year mark (Vizient, 2022). According to Vizient (2023), nurse residency programs' benefits to practice include the following:

- increased competency and confidence in clinical decision-making
- improved professional commitment
- job satisfaction and team interactions
- reduced turnover
- increased practice safety

Quality-of-care benefits include the following:

- improved quality and safety
- improved patient experience
- engaged and improved commitment of caregivers
- integrated organizational culture and values into nurses' practice

CASE STUDY 12.1

Julia is an emergency room nurse in a local critical access hospital in northern New England. She typically works 12-hour shifts, and during the height of the first and second surges of the COVID-19 virus, it was not unusual for Julia to work five to six 12-hour shifts per week. One evening, as she was driving home exhausted from work and saddened by the four patients who had died during her shift, she stopped at the grocery store to pick up bread and milk for her family. Upon exiting the store, she noticed that the front two tires of her car had been slashed, and she saw two young men running away from her car. When she yelled at them to stop, one of the young men turned and said, "You got what you deserved. You filled my mother with drugs that were poison and she died; COVID-19 didn't kill her—you and your medicine did!"

Julia was inconsolable, and when the police arrived to take her statement all she could say was, "Why don't they understand? Their mother wasn't vaccinated against the virus, and by the time she got to us it was too late?"

Workplace Health Amidst the COVID-19 Pandemic

Concerns for the health and safety of health care providers has always been a contributing factor to shortages. These concerns became even more magnified with the COVID-19 pandemic. Concerns include driving long distances to work and leaving family members and farm animals alone while at work, not knowing if they will return home because of the staffing shortages, working long hours, or even the possibility of contracting COVID or other infectious diseases while at work. Increases in workplace violence also contributed to concerns and fears for safety. More than 25% of nurses and other health care specialists in Australia work in rural settings. The risk factors these workers face include staffing shortages, extended shifts, frequent on-call responsibilities, high levels of stress, limited organizational support, and workplace violence (Franche et al., 2010). D. R. Terry et al. (2015) suggest that the needs are greater in rural areas due to significant intrinsic and extrinsic challenges, including poorer health outcomes and reduced life expectancies for rural dwellers.

The study participants comprised 15 public health nurses, including 13 women and two men, 40–60 years of age (D. R. Terry et al., 2015). Ten participants were from the northern region, three from the northwest Tasmanian region, one from the east coast and one from the west coast of Tasmania (D. R. Terry et al., 2015). The nurses had worked an average of 8.8 years, with the least experienced nurse working in a community setting for 3 years (see Table 12.1). This demographic data highlights the longevity of community health nurses who are viewed as "insiders" versus "outsiders" to their communities and therefore have both a personal and professional commitment to longevity in their roles.

TABLE 12.1 Demographics of Community Health Nurse Participants

Variable	n %
Sex (*n* = 15)	
Male	2 (13.3)
Female	13 (68.7)
Age groups, years (*n* = 15)	
30–39	1 (6.7)
40–49	3 (20.0)
50–59	10 (66.6)
60–65	1 (6.7)
Location of community health nurse (*n* = 15)	
In a large rural town	1 (6.7)
In a small rural town	12 (80.0)
Remote town	2 (13.3)
Years of experience in community health nursing (*n* = 15)	
1–5	1 (6.7)
6–10	2 (13.3)
10–15	4 (26.6)
16–20	2 (13.3)
21–25	1 (6.7)
26 or more	5 (33.4)

Source: D. R. Terry et al. (2015).

Data analysis of this study revealed multiple workplace health and safety issues (WHS) experienced by community health nurses (Terry et al., 2015). Multiple WHS themes were highlighted from the interview data, including geographic challenges and physical and environmental issues (Table 12.2). According to the researchers, experiential learning versus policies and procedures became the most important tool for these rural community health nurses, particularly in the area of overcoming violence. The researchers reported that "educating staff around violence and its negative consequences were highlighted, but rarely provided to staff" (Terry et al., 2015, p. 8). The researchers concluded that meeting the needs of community nurses was ultimately achieved, but these achievements were based on reactive versus proactive interventions to ensure the safety of the nurses and the rural dwellers in need of care.

TABLE 12.2 Themes Reported by Community Nurses

Themes	Subthemes	Clusters
Geographic environment issues	Driving large distances Working in isolation	Road conditions Travel times Weather Wildlife Lack of attention Personal safety Remoteness Poor phone reception Vulnerability
Physical environment issues	Client behavior Home condition Animals Smoking issues	Unpredictable clients Aggression and violence Poor home condition Fire hazard Clutter Poor bathrooms and beds Equipment risks working alone Aggressive animals Poor infection control Passion smoking
Organization/environment issues	Vertical and horizontal violence Workload, burnout, and work-related stress	Manager and staff violence Bullying Extremes of workload Documentation Dealing with the dying Dealing with client families

Source: D. R. Terry et al. (2015).

The Impact of Vaccine Hesitancy in Rural Areas

Mical et al. (2020) state that vaccine hesitancy is a pervading public health issue resulting in the delay or refusal of vaccines, which are known to offer protection against potentially deadly diseases. In 2017, the CDC documented an alarming increase in underimmunized children from 0.3% in 2001 to 1.3% in 2015 (CDC, 2018). In rural areas, these statistics indicate a significant health and safety threat. According to the CDC (2018), 100,000 children are unvaccinated against 14 potentially fatal diseases. Additionally, these numbers can be directly linked to increased compassion fatigue and caregiver burnout, increased emergency department visits, and morbidity and mortality rates (CDC, 2018; McClure et al., 2017). Mical et al. (2021) report that the 2019 measles outbreak afflicted primarily unvaccinated children in more than 31 states.

Professionally, nurses understand the science of vaccinations, but media misinformation and political influence changed all of that with the introduction of theories that question the effectiveness of the vaccine and potential adverse reactions. This evidence and the hesitancy surrounding the COVID-19 vaccine support the contribution of fear and resulting burnout for nurses as well as the urgency for more research into vaccine hesitancy, focusing on understanding the phenomenon, addressing barriers to action, and effective, culturally based strategies to eliminate this issue globally. During the COVID-19 pandemic, there were lower vaccination rates in rural areas with higher COVID-19 mortality rates (Sun & Monnat, 2021; Figures 12.2 and 12.3).

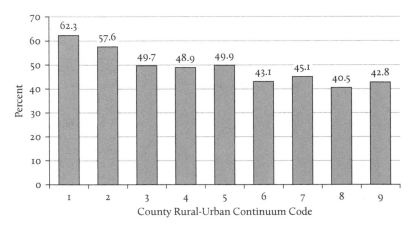

FIGURE 12.2 Percentage vaccination rate by rural-urban continuum code.

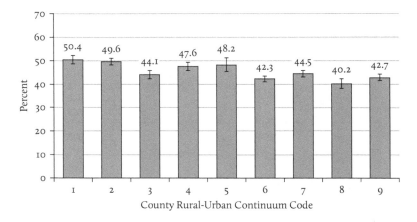

FIGURE 12.3 Average vaccination rate by rural-urban continuum code.

Conclusion

Many factors contributed to the sense of belonging among HCPs and nurses in particular, including increasing nurse burnout, fear of virus exposure and one's own health and safety, vaccine hesitancy among coworkers, and inconsistent practice standards. Nurses left the profession in record numbers, including those who were close to retirement age during the pandemic. Many cite a lack of support from administration, staffing shortages that resulted in unprecedented overtime hours, health and safety challenges, and political differences related to vaccinations. A review of data from the CDC (2021) confirms that COVID-19 vaccination rates are significantly lower in rural areas than in urban counties. Sun and Monnat (2021) state that "the largest contributors to lower rural vaccination rates are lower educational attainment and higher Trump vote share in the 2020 Presidential election" (Sun & Monnat, p. 916). Additionally, within rural counties, average vaccination rates are highest in recreation-dependent counties and lowest in mining and farming-dependent counties. This is concerning, given the high incidence of comorbidities that residents in these areas have that put their life expectancies at risk. Future planning must include strategies to provide information, education, and nursing care for workers in these areas that are vulnerable to new COVID-19 variants that could impact workplaces and rural workers who may be unvaccinated.

Addressing the vaccine crisis in rural areas will continue to require a multipronged approach. Sun and Monnat (2021) recommend that larger employers in rural communities hold regularly scheduled on-site vaccination clinics for employees and family members and provide employees with paid time off to get vaccinated and/or recover from any side effects. Other strategies in areas where the vaccine rates are higher should include educational opportunities sponsored by trusted community leaders to dispel misinformation regarding the COVID-19 vaccine and its risks. The National Rural Health Association (2023) has a plethora of free resources available for leaders to distribute and share on social media. Efforts based on a collaborative effort between nurses, primary care providers, and faith leaders that have an established level of trust with their communities may hold the best promise for a prevention strategy. It is also of value that standards of care and emergency protocols in times of high stress to HCPs and health care systems include responses to staffing shortages, support of nurses and other health care professionals, and clarification of expectations and job descriptions, regardless of reasons of higher demands on the health care system.

Questions for Discussion Related to Case Study 12.1

1. Does the case study highlight an example of workplace violence or vaccine hesitancy? Please elaborate on your response. Utilize information from the case to support your view.
2. Vaccine hesitancy is not uncommon in rural America. Why are rural communities more at risk for vaccine hesitancy? What can be done to mitigate these risks? Would these strategies necessitate changes in health care practices, health policies, or both?
3. How can the nursing and health care leadership in Julia's community support her and other nurses who may have been victimized because of misinformation regarding COVID-19 and vaccine hesitancy?

References

Centers for Disease Control and Prevention. (2018). *Vaccination coverage for selected diseases among children aged 19-35 months, by race, Hispanic origin, poverty level, and location of residence in metropolitan statistical areas: United States, selected years 1998-2017.* https://www.cdc.gov/mmwr/volumes/67/wr/mm6740a4.htm

Centers for Disease Control and Prevention. (2021). *COVID data tracker.* https://covid.cdc.gov/covid-data-tracker/#datatracker-home

Dos Santos, L. M. (2020). The relationship between the COVID-19 pandemic and nursing students' sense of belonging: The experiences and nursing education management of pre-service nursing professionals. *International Journal of Environmental Research and Public Health, 17*(5848), 1–18.

Farmer, J., Munoz, S., & Daly, C. (2012). Being rural in rural health research. *Health & Place, 18*, 1206–1208. https://doi.org/10.1016/j.healthplace.2012.05.002

Franche, R. L., Murray, E. J., Ostry, A., Ratner, P.A., Wagner S.L., Harder, H.G. (2010). Work disability prevention in rural areas: A focus on healthcare workers. *Rural Remote Health*, *10*, 1–24.

Goode, C. J., Glassman, K. S., Ponte, P. R., Krugman, M., & Peterson, T. (2018). Requiring a nurse residency for newly licensed nurses. *Nursing Outlook*, *66*(3), 329–332. https://doi.org/10.1016/j.outlook.2018.04.004

Knighten, M. L. (2022). New nurse residency programs: Benefits and return on investment. *Nursing Administration Quarterly*, *46*(2), 185–190. https://doi.org/10.1097/NAQ.0000000000000522

Levett-Jones, T., & Lathlean, J. (2008). Belongingness: A prerequisite for nursing students' clinical learning. *Nurse Education*, *8*(2), 103–111. https://www.proquest.com/scholarly-journals/staff-student-relationships-their-impact-on/docview/232493293/se-2?accountid=28932

Lockhart, L. (2020). Strategies to reduce nursing turnover. *Nursing Made Incredibly Easy*, *18*(2), 56.

Mical, R., Martin-Velez, J., Blackstone, T., & Derouin, A. (2021). Vaccine hesitancy in rural pediatric primary care. *Journal of Pediatric Health Care*, *35*(1), 16–22. https://doi.org/10.1016/j.pedhc.2020.07.003

McClure, C. C., Cataldi, J. R., & O'Leary, S. T. (2017). Vaccine hesitancy: Where are we and where are we going. *Clinical Therapeutics*, *39*, 1550–1562.

Mudallal, R. H., Othman, W. M., & Al Hassan, N. F. (2017). Nurses' burnout: The influence of leader empowering behaviors, work conditions, and demographic traits. *Inquiry: A Journal of Medical Care Organization, Provision and Financing*, *54*. https://doi.org/10.1177/0046958017724944

National Rural Health Association. (2023). *COVID-19 general resources*. https://www.rural-health.us/programs/covid-19-pandemic/covid-19-resources

Ross, A. (February 16, 2021). *Maine's rural hospitals in crisis, now asking lawmakers for more relief*. WMTW News 8. https://www.wmtw.com/article/maines-rural-hospitals-in-crisis-now-asking-lawmakers-for-more-relief/35525782#

Sablik, T. (2022). The rural nursing shortage. *Econ Focus*, *27*(1), 4–7.

Sellers, K., Riley, M., Denny, D., Rogers, D., Havener, J.-M., Rathbone, T., & Cesare, C. G.-D. (2019). Retention of nurses in a rural environment: The impact of job satisfaction, resilience, grit, engagement, and rural fit. *Online Journal of Rural Nursing and Health Care*, *19*(1), 4–42. https://doi.org/10.14574/ojrnhc.v19i1.547

Sharp, D. B. (2010). *Factors related to the recruitment and retention of nurse practitioners in rural areas* [PhD dissertation, The University of Texas at El Paso] (3409167). ProQuest Dissertations & Theses Global. https://www.proquest.com/dissertations-theses/factors-related-recruitment-retention-nurse/docview/613695577/se-2

Short, K., Freedman, K., Matays, J., Rosamilia, M., Wade, K., (2019). Making the transition: A critical care skills program to support newly hired nurses. *Clinical. Nurse Specialist*, *33*(3), 123-127. https://doi.org/10.1097/NUR.0000000000000444

Smith, S., Lapkin, S., Halcomb, E., & Sim, J. (2023). Job satisfaction among small rural hospital nurses: A cross-sectional study. *Journal of Nursing Scholarship*, *55*(1), 378–387. https://doi.org/10.1111/jnu.12800

Sun, Y., & Monnat, S. M. (2022). Rural-urban and within-rural differences in COVID-19 vaccination rates. *The Journal of Rural Health: Official Journal of the American Rural Health Association and the National Rural Health Care Association*, *38*(4), 916–922. https://doi.org/10.1111/jrh.12625

Terry, D., Lê, Q., Nguyen, U., & Ha, H. (2015). Workplace health and safety issues among community nurses: A study regarding the impact on providing care to rural consumers. *BMJ Open*, *5*(8), 1–10. https://doi.org/10.1136/bmjopen-2015-008306

Terry, D. R., Lê, Q., Hoang, H., & Barrett, A. (2015). Rural community nurses: Insights into health workforce and health service needs in Tasmania. *International Journal of Health, Wellness & Society, 5*(3), 109–120. https://doi.org/10.18848/2156-8960/CGP/v05i03/58094

Ulrich, B., Krozek, C., Early, S., Ashlock, C. H., Africa, L. M., & Carman, M. L. (2010). Improving retention, confidence, and competence of new graduate nurses: Results from a 10-year longitudinal database. *Nursing Economics, 28*(6), 363–375.

U.S. Department of Health and Human Services, Health Resources and Services Administration. (2010). *The registered nurse population: Findings from the 2008 national sample survey of registered nurses. https://data.hrsa.gov/DataDownload/NSSRN/GeneralPUF08/rnsurveyfinal.pdf*

U.S. Department of Health and Human Services, Health Resources and Services Administration (2017, July 21). *Supply and demand projections of the nursing workforce: 2014-20130.* https://bhw.hrsa.gov/sites/default/files/bureau-health-workforce-data-research/nchwa-hrsa-nursing-report.pdf

Vizient. (2022). *Nurturing a better nurse: The case for a nurse residency program.* https://www.vizientinc.com/-/media/documents/sitecorepublishingdocuments/public/nurturing-abetternurse.pdf

Vizient. (2023). *What is the Vizient/AACN Nurse Residency Program?* https://www.vizientinc.com/what-we-do/operations-and-quality/vizient-aacn-nurse-residency-program

Wakefield, E., Innes, K., Dix, S., & Brand, G. (2023). Belonging in high acuity settings: What is needed for newly graduated registered nurses to successfully transition? A qualitative systematic review. *Nurse Education Today, 121.* https://doi.org/10.1016/j.nedt.2022.105686

Walker, L., Clendon, J., & Willis, J. (2018). Why older nurses leave the profession. *Kai Tiaki Nursing Research, 9*(1), 5–11.

Willis, E., Reynolds, L., & Keleher, H. (2019). *Understanding the Australian health care system.* Elsevier.

Image Credits

Fig. 12.1: Source: https://www.richmondfed.org/publications/research/econ_focus/2022/q1_feature_1.

Fig. 12.2: Source: Yue Sun and Shannon M. Monnat, "Rural-Urban and Within-Rural Differences in COVID-19 Vaccination Rates," The Journal of Rural Health, https://onlinelibrary.wiley.com/doi/10.1111/jrh.12625, 2021.

Fig. 12.3: Source: Yue Sun and Shannon M. Monnat, "Rural-Urban and Within-Rural Differences in COVID-19 Vaccination Rates," The Journal of Rural Health, https://onlinelibrary.wiley.com/doi/10.1111/jrh.12625, 2021.

CHAPTER 13

Preparing for Nursing Practice During a Global Pandemic

Al-Taweel et al. (2020) stated that during the COVID-19 pandemic, academic institutions worldwide were not adequately prepared to address education: "Whether they are novices or experts ... the instant shift to online platforms did not allow many to be well prepared for the challenges ahead" (p. 1296). According to the researchers, when the government shutdowns moved education from on-campus to "in-house" teaching and learning, many students were not in a situation to interact with health care team members to develop this sense of belonging to something greater (Al-Taweel et al., 2020).

In early spring of 2020, shifting to online modalities of nursing education became an emergent issue for nursing colleges and universities across the United States. Many programs scrambled to set up online learning platforms that allowed students to engage in real-time education while adhering to governmental restrictions to slow the spread of the COVID-19 virus. This was less of a seismic shift for some programs than for others. Larger, urban universities typically offer a blend of on-ground and online instruction for nursing students. Didactic learning can occur synchronously under a faculty member's guidance or asynchronously. Asynchronous learning in nursing typically involves faculty creating content placed within an online platform for learners to progress through their program and prepare for the National Council of State Boards of Nursing (NCSBN) registered nurse licensing exam (NCLEX). This technology is costly and depends on reliable broadband connections, which are often lacking in many rural settings. A common learning modality for students in rural and remote regions remains face-to-face classroom learning. Hodges et al. (2020) state that emergency remote teaching in many areas offered online education in the absence of thoughtful and sustainable plans for learning. As we emerge from the pandemic, it is important to examine the issues surrounding nursing practice and education so we can learn from these experiences and build strategic plans for the future of nursing education.

Critical Information and Competencies for Entry Into Nursing Practice

In 2020, the WHO stated that the focus of education for nurses preparing for entry into practice should be on the delivery of patient-centered care, "ensuring the quality of care and patient safety, preventing and controlling infections, and combating antimicrobial resistance" (p. 12). The WHO (2020) suggests that the nurse's role should prioritize health promotion, health literacy, and management of noncommunicable diseases. Lastly, the WHO also emphasizes that nursing education programs must prepare students for their critical role in the management of epidemics, irrespective of educational level. However, nursing faculty have expressed concerns regarding the overwhelming amount of content that is already in undergraduate curricula, and many educators have expressed concerns about further overwhelming learners with content that is not heavily tested on the NCLEX examination (Morin, 2020). Proponents of change argue that given the circumstances and crises by managing nursing education programs, the focus of curricula should be modified so that content on disaster preparedness and emergency and pandemic responses can be included. Additionally, a shift in program content could allow for the inclusion of more information on the social determinants of health, caring for persons with noncommunicable diseases, and the role of the nurse in preserving planetary health (Morin, 2020).

The Essentials: Core Competencies for Professional Nursing Education

The COVID-19 pandemic has provided nursing leaders with evidence regarding the need for a dramatic shift in nursing education, particularly at the entry-to-practice level. The focus of this change will require refocusing undergraduate nursing curricula to include content that supports building graduates' knowledge, skills, and attitudes to function as competent and confident nurse generalists. Morin (2020) states, "Although the care of mothers, infants, and children is considered essential undergraduate knowledge in most countries, one could argue that this information would be more appropriately placed at a postgraduate program level" (p. 3118). These changes would reinforce the AACN's (2021) core competencies for professional nursing education.

The Implications of the COVID-19 Pandemic for Nursing Education

Badowski et al. (2021) researched the implications of the COVID-19 pandemic on nursing education and presented recommendations for changes to nursing curricula based on surveys of frontline nurses during the first wave of the pandemic. The researchers recruited nurses throughout the United States ($n = 100$) to complete the study protocol. Table 13.1 details the diversity of the study sample.

TABLE 13.1 Diversity of Frontline Nurses Surveyed During Initial Wave of the COVID-19 Pandemic

Race	Percent of Study Sample
White	37%
Black	20%
Latinx	20%
Asian	14%
Multiracial	7%
Native American	2%
Transgender and nonbinary	2%

Source: Badowski et al. (2021).

Nursing Practice Recommendations

The 100 study participants articulated that nursing leaders must emphasize four themes: (a) teamwork and communication, (b) flexibility and critical thinking, (c) leadership and using your voice, and (d) advocacy and policy. Badowski et al. (2021) stated that the shift to heightened importance on the interpersonal skills nurses must possess reflects a paradigm shift that presents a new challenge in nursing education. This shift is congruent with the findings of a review conducted by Theisen and Sandau (2013), who looked at 26 unique studies and discovered a lack of critical thinking and communication skills among new nurses. In light of the events that transpired during the height of the COVID-19 pandemic, this critical study should be replicated and focus on new graduates during the post-COVID-19 era to assess these concerns in greater detail (Badowski et al., 2021).

Nurse educators should design continuing education offerings that focus on these themes to equip new graduates with the knowledge and skills they will need to best prepare and retain these nurses in hospitals, community health centers, ambulatory care settings, and urban medical centers.

CASE STUDY 13.1

Amy is a registered nurse who just received notice that she has been conditionally hired at an acute care rural hospital in the northeastern United States. Amy is scheduled to sit for her NCLEX licensure examination in 3 weeks, and she has been studying for the exam and answering practice questions on a daily basis. One afternoon, Amy stops at the grocery store to get a supply of snacks she and her friend can eat during their evening study session. As she approaches the checkout registers, she sees two nurses in scrubs and overhears a troubling conversation. One nurse states, "Did you hear we are getting another new graduate next week?" Her colleague responds, "Oh gosh, not another one who has more experience caring for mannequins than real patients!" As she exits the checkout line, Amy can feel the tears forming in her eyes. Later that evening she shares the experience with her friend and states, "What are we doing? Are we kidding ourselves, or are we really ready to take care of patients?"

Teamwork and Communication

In Badowski et al.'s (2021) study, frontline bedside nurses during the first wave of the COVID-19 pandemic in the United States described teamwork and communication as primary themes needed in nursing education. The participants defined *communication* as a team process that may occur during bedside care or remotely among nurses, patients, and other health care providers to share feelings, education, information, or ideas. Participants emphasized the collegiality that occurred among nurses and providers of care and how that translated to the highest quality of patient care.

Flexibility and Critical Thinking

Critical thinking was described as a process used to investigate potential options utilized to determine priorities in an active and systematized way that is self-directed, self-regulated, and self-corrective (Badowski et al., 2021). According to participant responses, nursing education should ideally aim to assist students to learn flexibility and critical thinking related to the dynamic nature of health care. One participant stated, "Nurses should come out with the ability to think critically. I don't think the technical skills are what's most important, but the ability to think through the processes" (Badowski et al., 2021, p. 671).

Leadership and Using Your Voice

Leadership in the Badowski et al. (2021) study was defined as a process that can occur during face-to-face encounters or remotely when a nurse provides information, support, and education to an individual or a group of individuals to achieve specific goals in the provision of nursing care and in the nursing profession. One participant stated, "Stand up for yourself from a ... leadership perspective. ... You bring value to the table ... Communicate your needs." Another participant stated that nurses must remember to use their nursing education and judgment to guide consumers of health care in a direction that will allow them to make safe choices (Badowski et al., 2021, p. 671).

Advocacy and Health Policy

The participants stressed the importance of nurses using their voices outside of work settings as community and public policy advocates. One participant stated, "Look at how we address our health care in low-income communities. ... We need to look at how we are providing care" (Badowski et al., 2021, p. 671). The study participants also emphasized the importance of educating nursing students about the relationship between policy decisions and their impact on patient care.

Finding a New Normal for Nursing Education and Practice

Barton et al. (2020) stated in an open letter to nurse educators that the new normal resulting from the COVID-19 pandemic is desperately needed changes in the content and delivery modalities for nursing curricula: "Nursing education programs that have not been traditionally included in nursing education's embrace of online and remote learning, such as accelerated baccalaureate nursing degrees and many types of graduate programs, have successfully made these transitions" (p. 183). Nurse educators must now innovate the assessment and evaluation practices for these programs.

Giddens (2020) states that the trend of competency-based nursing education is evolving and will continue to be widely supported by the AACN (2021). Giddens (2020) advises nursing faculty members to embrace and become more familiar with concept-based and competency approaches to nursing education: "Concepts represent the cognitive structures for students to organize their thinking and learning" (p. 123). "Competencies provide a standard, intentional approach for learner assessment that can validate competence in that area" (Giddens, 2020, p. 124). Nursing educators must acknowledge this approach for students as we proceed into postpandemic practice and begin to intentionally prepare for future emergencies that may require students to enter practice quickly and seamlessly as competent and confident providers of care.

Use of Simulation for Preparing Students

Not only were real-life clinical settings limited in rural settings, but they became nonexistent with the pandemic. Many health care students began to participate in clinical experiences in a virtual simulation situation (Fogg et al., 2020). *Virtual simulation* is best defined as a screen-based experience that is partially immersive and allows one to observe and interact in various opportunities (Shin & Rim, 2023). A systematic review by Foronda et al. (2020) indicated that virtual simulation was an effective pedagogy to support learning outcomes. However, there have always been concerns as well as limitations for the number of clinical hours students receive as compared to actual interactive clinical situations.

For undergraduate nursing programs, the NCSBN (2016) recommends the use of simulation as a substitution for clinical experiences but not to exceed 50% of the programs' total clinical hours. Many research studies have been conducted over the past decade examining the benefits of integrating simulation and virtual learning programs into nursing education. Kim et al. (2016) designed a meta-analysis study that described a medium-to-large effect size (0.70), suggesting the effectiveness of integrating simulation-based learning (SBL) in nursing education. Curl et al. (2016) conducted a study involving the replacement of on-ground clinical experiences with simulation for prelicensure nursing students. Findings from the study indicated significantly higher scores for students on the pregraduation exit examination than traditional clinical experiences alone.

Kimhi et al. (2016) designed a double-crossover study examining the differences in self-confidence and self-efficacy between two groups of nursing students enrolled in a nursing program in Israel. The majority of both groups of students were single women with a mean age of 23.5 years (Kimhi et al., 2016). Findings from this research indicated that students' self-confidence/self-efficacy was increased following both clinical experience and simulations that focused on the nursing process. However, the influence of the clinical experience was stronger. In 2020, a waiver was issued in the state of Texas that permitted senior nursing students in their final program year to meet clinical learning objectives by exceeding the 50% limit on clinical simulation learning experiences (Texas Board of Nursing, 2020). The passage of the waiver had several aims. First, to minimize the interruption that nursing students were experiencing due to the sudden restrictions in health care organizations students were assigned to for clinical learning experiences. Additionally, the waiver allowed students in their final year minimal interruption in their programs so that they could complete the clinical requirements, enter nursing practice, and provide care for the growing numbers of patients presenting with dire symptoms of COVID-19.

Graduate students were also impacted by the closure of hospitals and health care organizations. Faculty scrambled to support these students who were required to meet the mandated clinical hours. Graduate students who are enrolled in APRN programs in the state of Texas must complete a clinical practicum or preceptorship to complete their program, allowing them the opportunity to provide direct patient care under the supervision of experienced faculty members and preceptors (Texas Board of Nursing, 2013). For graduate students, "The state waiver increasing the limit of simulation hours only applied to course-related clinical hours in excess of the minimum standard direct care hours (500 hours) required by the Texas Board of Nursing" (Fogg et al., 2020, p. 686).

In order to examine the challenges and opportunities of on-ground clinical learning and learning through virtual simulation, researchers surveyed undergraduate and graduate students using a 5-point Likert scale to determine the transition from traditional clinical learning to virtual clinical experiences (Fogg et al., 2020). Fifty-three percent of the undergraduate students surveyed agreed or strongly agreed that virtual simulation experiences provided valuable opportunities that strengthened their learning. Twenty-one percent were neutral, and 12% responded negatively. The remaining 14% selected not applicable (NA), which may account for students who were not enrolled in a clinical course during that time (Fogg et al., 2020).

In the qualitative responses, students were open about the challenges they faced during the pandemic, which included internet connection, the inability to log onto web conferencing, family distractions, and inexperience of clinical faculty who were required to teach in an online environment. However, the overall response from students was positive and noted "appreciation for quickly developing a transition plan to virtual learning as a replacement for clinical learning experiences, support for students to support program progression and on-time graduation" (Fogg et al., 2020, p. 690).

Graduate students expressed their overall satisfaction of the virtual learning experiences after the on-ground clinical sites were closed during the height of the COVID-19 pandemic. The modified curriculum allowed most students to complete all their required clinical hours. The presentation of case studies were viewed more positively and preferred by many students over telemedicine. However, despite the overall positive feedback, graduate students reported that their existing high stress levels, which they attributed to being in a graduate program, were worsened by the academic and personal changes that occurred during the height of the pandemic (Fogg et al., 2020).

Fogg et al. (2020) stated that for both undergraduate and graduate students, there were several restrictive factors that impacted faculty members' ability to deliver clinical experiences and students' ability to assimilate those experiences, including clinical agency restrictions, the requirements of licensing and accrediting bodies, and the access to and use of technology to deliver virtual learning experiences. Each of these factors must be addressed collaboratively between nursing programs and health care organizations. These collaborations could increase APRN clinical learning, including experiences managing health care needs that arise during a pandemic or natural disaster.

International Updates on the Use of Simulation

Nursing researchers have conducted few single-center related studies on the use of simulation and clinical learning in nursing. Alshutwi et al. (2022) aimed to articulate the efficacy and effectiveness of SBL as a substitute for all clinical training in all nursing courses.

Additionally, they aimed to investigate the association between SBL effectiveness and students' demographic characteristics. The study was designed as a cross-sectional descriptive survey that asked for participants' responses on their perceptions regarding the effectiveness of SBL. A convenience sample of 375 students were emailed the electronic self-report surveys, and 308 students completed and returned the surveys. The Modified Simulation Effectiveness Tool (SET-M), a tool developed in 2005 that includes a prebriefing subscale, a scenario subscale, and a 5-item debriefing subscale, was used for data collection with overall internal consistency. A higher score of the tool reflects students' favorable perceptions of the simulation (Alshutwi et al., 2022).

Findings from this research indicated that most students agreed that the prebriefing improved both their learning and self-confidence (Alshutwi et al., 2022). Additionally, students stated that debriefing was beneficial to their learning because it allowed them to verbalize their feelings, enhance their clinical judgment, improve self-reflection, and build a constructive self-evaluation. The researchers stated that this study could add to the body of evidence-based knowledge regarding the effect of SBL on students' knowledge, self-efficacy, and confidence.

The Impact of the COVID-19 Pandemic on the Lives and Learning Experiences of Nursing Students

The COVID-19 pandemic resulted in a global shift to online, distance learning modalities for nursing and other health care students. These changes resulted in the role of students going from passive learners to active participants in their education (Posey & Pintz, 2017; Sharples et al., 2016). Many students were physically displaced from their familiar classroom and clinical learning environments and relocated back to their residence, which often posed a barrier to distance learning, whether in the form of limited internet resources or an atmosphere not conducive to learning or a supportive environment, and "not being able to be present in clinical settings makes students feel that they are missing out on a golden opportunity to acquire skills and enhancing doubt and uncertainty" (Masha'al et al., 2020 p. 671).

Masha'al et al. (2020) conducted a qualitative study with participants from Jordan that indicated students' abilities to manage these uncertainties was directly influenced by their socioeconomic characteristics and revealed four themes as the main sources of stress: unorganized workloads, lack of a standardized distance learning strategy, limited resources, and distracting environments.

The students who came from low socioeconomic environments experienced the highest levels of stress, namely unorganized workloads, lacked a standardized distance learning strategy, had limited resources, and were in distracting environments. These factors should be the focus of faculty and student debriefing sessions so that changes in universities policies and legislative policies can be designed and implemented proactively to support students who are living and learning through future public health emergencies.

Conclusion

Haslam (2021) stated that the move to accept online and hybrid models of nursing education has been inevitable for decades. However, the COVID-19 pandemic accelerated the speed of these changes. The benefits of online learning allows a larger number of nursing students to choose learning modalities that eliminate time-based and geographic boundaries. If nursing programs are offered in varied modalities there will be increased student enrollment in these programs as a result of the diversity and inclusivity of varied learning strategies that are available through online and hybrid learning options. These innovations may be a positive first step to addressing the global nursing shortage. However, these changes may pose challenges for other learners who are more comfortable in a traditional, on-ground classroom setting.

Questions for Discussion Related to Case Study 13.1

1. What does the literature report regarding the preparedness of students who were educated since the beginning of the COVID-19 pandemic? Does the data reflect both competence and confidence in nursing practice in these graduates compared to graduates prior to the start of the pandemic?
2. Should employers provide unique support for recent graduates, such as extended orientation programs or support networks in which these nurses can feel free to express their worries regarding transitioning into nursing practice?
3. Should nursing education leaders modify current curricula at all levels of practice and infuse education that is focused on natural disasters and public health emergencies to proactively plan for future crises? Should this education be evident on future versions of the NCLEX examination?

References

Alshutwi, S., Alsharif, F., Shibily, F., Wedad M, A., Almotairy, M. M., & Algabbashi, M. (2022). Maintaining Clinical training continuity during COVID-19 pandemic: Nursing students' perceptions about simulation-based learning. *International Journal of Environmental Research and Public Health, 19*(4), 2180. https://doi.org/10.3390/ijerph19042180

Al-Taweel, D., Al-Hagan, A., Bajis, D., Al-Bader, J., Al-Taweel, A. R., Al-Awadhi, A., & Al-Awadhi, F. (2020). Multidisciplinary academic perspectives during COVID-19 pandemic. *International Journal of Health Planning Management, 35*(6), 1–7.

American Association of Colleges of Nursing. (2021). *The essentials: Core competencies for professional nursing education*. https://www.aacnnursing.org/essentials

Badowski, D. M., Spurlark, R., Webber-Ritchey, K., Towson, S., Ponder, T. N., & Simonovich, S. D. (2021). Envisioning nursing education for a post–COVID-19 world: Qualitative findings from the frontline. *Journal of Nursing Education, 60*(12), 668–673. https://doi.org/10.3928/01484834-20211004-03

Barton, A. J., Murray, T. A., & Spurlock, D. R. (2020). An open letter to members of the nursing education community. *Journal of Nursing Education, 59*(4), 183. https://doi.org/10.3928/01484834-20200323-01

Curl, E. D., Smith, S., Chisholm, L. A., McGee, L. A. & Das, K. (2016). Effectiveness of integrated simulation and clinical experiences compared to traditional clinical experiences for nursing students. *Nursing Education Perspectives, 37*(2), 72–77. https://doi.org/10.5480/15-1647

Fogg, N., Wilson, C., Trinka, M., Campbell, R., Thomson, A., Merritt, L., Tietze, M., & Prior, M. (2020). Transitioning from direct care to virtual clinical experiences during the COVID-19 pandemic. *Journal of Professional Nursing, 36*(6), 685–691. https://doi.org/10.1016/j.profnurs.2020.09.012

Foronda, C. L., Fernandez-Burgos, M., Nadeau, C. Kelley, C. N., & Henry, M. N. (2020). Virtual simulation in nursing education: A systematic review spanning 1996 to 2018. *Simulation in Healthcare: Journal of the Society for Medical Simulation, 15*(1), 46–54. https://doi.org/10.1097/SIH.0000000000000411

Giddens, J. (2020). Demystifying concept-based and competency-based approaches. *Journal of Nursing Education, 59*(3), 123–124. https://doi.org/10.3928/01484834-20200220-01

Haslam, M. B. (2021). What might COVID-19 have taught us about the delivery of nurse education, in a post-COVID-19 world? *Nurse Education Today, 97*, 104707. https://doi.org/10.1016/j.nedt.2020.104707

Hodges, C., Moore, S., Lockee, B., Trust, T., & Bond, A. (2020, March 27). The difference between emergency remote teaching and online learning. *EDUCAUSE Review.* https://link.springer.com/chapter/10.1007/978-981-15-7869-4_3

Kim, J., Park, J.-H., & Shin, S. (2016). Effectiveness of simulation-based nursing education depending on fidelity: A meta-analysis. *BMC Medical Education, 16*(152), 1–8. https://doi.org/10.1186/s12909-016-0672-7

Kimhi, E., Reishtein, J. L., Cohen, M., Friger, M., Hurvitz, N., & Avraham, R. (2016). Impact of simulation and clinical experience on self-efficacy in nursing students. *Nurse Educator, 41*(1), E1–E4. https://doi.org/10.1097/NNE.0000000000000194

Masha'al, D., Rababa, M., & Shahrour, G. (2020). Distance learning–related stress among undergraduate nursing students during the COVID-19 pandemic. *Journal of Nursing Education, 59*(12), 666–674. https://doi.org/10.3928/01484834-20201118-03

Morin, K. H. (2020). Nursing education after COVID-19: Same or different? *Journal of Clinical Nursing, 29*(17–18), 3117–3119. https://doi.org/10.1111/jocn.15322

National Council of State Boards of Nursing. (2016). *Simulation guidelines for prelicensure nursing education programs.* https://www.ncsbn.org/public-files/16_Simulation_Guidelines.pdf

Posey, L., & Pintz, C. (2017). Transitioning a Bachelor of Science in nursing program to blended learning: Successes, challenges & outcomes. *Nurse Education in Practice, 26*, 126–133. https://doi.org/10.1016/j.nepr.2016.10.006

Sharples, M., de Roock, R., Ferguson, R., Gaved, M., Herodotou, C., Koh, E., Kukulska-Hulme, A., Looi, C. K., McAndrew, P., Rienties, B., Weller, M., & Wong, L. H. (2016). *Innovating pedagogy 2016: Open University innovation report 5.* Institute of Educational Technology, The Open University.

Shin, H., & Rim, D. (2023). Development and assessment of a curriculum model for virtual simulation in nursing: Curriculum development and pilot-evaluation. *BMC Med Education, 23*(1), 284. doi.org/10.1186/s12909-023-04283-4

Texas Board of Nursing. (2013). *APRN education requirements for licensure.* https://www.bon.texas.gov/applications_advanced_practice_registered_nurse.asp.html

Theisen, J. L., & Sandau, K. E. (2013). Competency of new graduate nurses: A review of their weaknesses and strategies for success. *The Journal of Continuing Education in Nursing, 44*(9), 406–414. https://doi.org/10.3928/00220124-20130617-38

World Health Organization. (2020). *State of the world's nursing: Investing in education, jobs and leadership.* https://www.who.int/publications/i/item/9789240003279

CHAPTER 14

The Challenges and Opportunities of Entering Practice During a Global Pandemic

C linical settings immediately discontinued access for students when it was apparent that COVID-19 was extremely contagious, limiting opportunities for students to experience hands-on care. This limitation was even more acute in rural health care settings where clinical sites are more scarce. Nonrural settings include urban and metropolitan hospitals, other inpatient facilities, emergency departments, hospital-sponsored ambulatory care facilities, nursing homes and long-term care facilities, correctional institutions, private medical care practices, school health clinics, urgent care services, occupational health settings, university/college health clinics, and home health agencies (Stellflug et al., 2022). One rural community may provide a critical access hospital (CAH) setting that includes a long-term care facility and an emergency department only. Many CAHs in remote areas do not even have acute beds; their goal is to stabilize and transfer. Current literature indicates that if health care students have exposure to rural and remote settings, there is a possibility that they will choose to return to that setting for employment upon graduation, thus addressing health care provider shortages in rural communities (Buerhaus et al., 2015). With no exposure to rural health care settings for these students, the shortage of health care staff, including nurses, grew even more acute.

Transition to Nursing Practice Amidst a Global Pandemic

The COVID-19 pandemic had a global effect on all levels of nursing education. Senior nursing students preparing for graduation and entering practice and employment were particularly impacted by the events of the pandemic as they desperately tried to complete didactic and clinical degree requirements. The complexities involved in transitioning to practice are described by Meleis (2010) as a process that demonstrates understanding and acceptance of change as a part of the nurse's new responsibilities. For many nursing graduates, there are a multitude of questions that must be answered:

- Do I have the skills that will be required to be successful in my new role?
- Will I be able to find mentoring support from my new colleagues, particularly if a formal mentoring program does not exist?
- How will I effectively navigate communicating with nursing and health care leaders in my new place of employment?

These issues were compounded by the events of the COVID-19 pandemic, which had wide-ranging impacts on nursing graduates' transition to practice. Phillips et al. (2023) examined clinical faculty members' and preceptors' assessment of senior nursing students' strengths in practice and challenges as compared to those of graduates of years prior to the onset of the COVID-19 pandemic. Faculty from two colleges in the United States participated in an online Qualtrics survey starting in May 2021 that asked questions related to graduates' eight clinical competencies. Table 14.1 provides a comparison of study respondents' ($n = 19$) evaluation of competencies of senior nursing students graduating in 2021 and prior year graduates (PYGs).

A rating of level 1, indicating not met, was used one time by one study participant for professionalism and one time by one participant under the category evidence-based practice for the 2021 graduates only. However, all other respondents rated the PYG and 2021 graduates as either *met* or *exceeded* in all categories. It is important to note that there were significant differences in the ratings of students based on their year of graduation in four categories: evidence-based practice ($p = .009$), safety ($p = .011$), informatics ($p = .012$), and professionalism ($p = .038$) (Phillips et al., 2023).

TABLE 14.1 Clinical Simulation Competency Assessment Tool Results

Competency	2021	2021	2021	PYG	PYG	PYG	X_2
	Not Met	Met	Exceeded	Not Met	Met	Exceeded	
Patient-centered care	0%	52.6%	47.4%	0%	15.8%	84.2%	$X_2 = 3.206$, $p = .073$
Teamwork and collaboration	0%	57.9%	42.1%	0%	36.8%	63.2%	$X_2 = 3.519$ $p = .061$
Evidence-based practice	0%	57.9%	42.1%	0%	47.4%	52.6%	$X_2 = 6.739$, $p = .055$
Quality improvement	0%	78.9%	21.1%	0%	42.1%	57.9%	$X_2 = 3.685$, $p = .055$
Safety	0%	42.1%	57.9%	0%	21.1%	78.9%	$X_2 = 6.429$, $p = .011*$
Informatics	0%	68.4%	31.6%	0%	42.1%	57.9%	$X_2 = 6.378$, $p = .012*$
Professionalism	5.3%	31.6%	63.2%	0%	21.1%	78.9%	$X_2 = 6.537$, $p = .038*$
System-based practice	5.3%	57.9%	36.8%	0%	42.1%	57.9%	$X_2 = 4.296$, $p = .117$

Data analysis focusing on the qualitative responses from study participants reflect a range of strengths and barriers from the COVID-19 pandemic, but there was no consistent pattern and some disagreement among respondents. The majority of respondents did acknowledge the notion of "support," which included changes hospitals and nursing programs could and should make to connect with students and their needs and interventions that nursing professional development specialists and nurses at the bedside that, as a whole, could be more helpful to new graduates transitioning to professional practice (Phillips et al., 2023).

CASE STUDY 14.1

Jacob is a registered nurse who was hired 10 weeks ago as a float nurse in a critical access hospital located in a rural community in Kentucky. Jacob has always prided himself as a fast learner, and he was the top graduate of his second-degree baccalaureate class at the state's largest academic institution. Jacob had been offered other positions in urban hospitals, but he chose to go back to the community where his family and aging parents reside. This morning, Jacob cared for a patient who died of complications related to the COVID-19 virus. When Jenna, the nurse manager, enters the nurse's station where Jacob is writing his final note for the deceased patient, she overhears him talking with another nurse who is trying to comfort him. Jacob states, "Maybe Jim would still be here if I were more skilled to manage his needs. Honestly, the more shifts I work, the more I doubt my ability to provide care." Jacob's colleague attempts to provide words of encouragement, but she too is overwhelmed with patient care needs and her advice to him is "Recognize that we are all trying to manage this crisis as best as we can, you with little help and resources."

Jenna returns to her office both saddened and concerned about Jacob and the 10 other new graduates who have left the hospital since the beginning of the pandemic. Jenna shares this with a nurse manager on another unit who expresses agreement and asks Jenna if she would be interested in creating a nurse residency program. Jenna and her colleague are determined to look for solutions regardless of the limitations of staff and other resources.

The Impact on NCLEX Scores

In early 2020, the forced and abrupt closure of many nursing programs resulted in faculty members and nursing leaders shifting to virtual and online modalities of learning. These shifts left many faculty members with concerns regarding their students' abilities to be successful on the National Council Licensure Examination (NCLEX). In March 2020, faculty at Georgia College & State University looked at faculty and student surveys as well as standardized exit examinations and NCLEX-RN pass rates to determine the usefulness of virtual simulation instead of traditional bedside clinical experiences during the final semester of a prelicensure baccalaureate program (Roberts et al., 2022). Findings from the research are indicative of a slight decrease in exit exam scores as compared to those who completed traditional clinical experiences and had no significant relationship between NCLEX-RN pass/fail rates.

The National Council of State Boards of Nursing (NCSBN) works with state boards of nursing to regulate nursing practice: Nursing regulatory boards protect the public's health and welfare by assuring "safe and competent nursing care is provided through regulation, practice and education" (NCSBN, 2024, Nursing Regulation section). The NCSBN, which reports NCLEX pass rates yearly, noted a decrease in the NCLEX pass rates since the start of the pandemic, indicating the impact of the changes made to educational programs in response to the COVID-19 crisis (Table 14.2).

TABLE 14.2 NCLEX Pass Rates Through the Pandemic

Degree	2019	2020	2021	2022
Diploma	87.89	86.33	79.53	79.18
Baccalaureate	91.22	90.29	86.06	82.95
Associate	85.17	82.80	78.78	78.92

Source: Wenxia et al. (2022).

The Impact of COVID-19 on Preceptorships and Residencies

As an attempt to retain graduate nurses transitioning into practicing, many facilities have implemented nurse residencies and preceptorships, especially in urban settings. Transition shock occurs when a graduate nurse transitions into a practicing professional with changes in responsibilities, roles, relationships, and environment that result in stressors that include feelings of uncertainty and confusion that can lead to job dissatisfaction.

Multiple factors associated with transition shock influence the type of transition to practice (TTP) that new graduates will experience. Preceptorships offer unique learning opportunities and support to graduates to navigate through their TTP. Often faculty will encourage graduate nurses to seek employment with systems that provide preceptorships and residencies and to ask questions regarding the quality, training, and length of any preceptorship program that might be of interest to their professional development. However, nurse residencies and preceptors can be limited in rural health care settings. One solution to this issue might be found in the National Rural Recruitment and Retention Network (3RNET). This is a nonprofit network funded by the Federal Office of Rural Health Policy and one of the largest and most comprehensive recruitment and retention resources in the U.S. (Rural Health Information Hub, 2022). Member organizations include community health centers, hospitals, private practices, and community-based organizations. These organization can post job openings that can be easily retrieved by health care workers seeking employment (Rural Health Information Hub, 2022). Baldwin et al. (2021) stated that graduate nurses value preceptors' positivity, patience, and advocacy on their behalf and struggle when they are impatient, have unrealistic expectations, or display incivility. According to Edwards et al. (2015), genuine support and concern from experienced nurse preceptors and experienced nurses while a graduate is committed to a residency are essential for a successful transition. Wenxia et al. (2022) also add that nursing management can reduce transition shock by creating a friendly and supportive environment and addressing feedback-seeking behavior in new nurses. Smith et al. (2021) also confirmed that an open and collegial learning environment facilitated effective TTP.

Unionization

During and after the pandemic, nurse staffing shortages became even more acute with increased patient census and challenging patients of high acuity. When a facility is under-staffed, the quality of patient care can be compromised. Routine care that many patients expected just could not possibly be provided (Davidson, 2023). As a result, many patients and their family members became frustrated with care providers. This frustration set up many facilities and providers for increased workplace violence. Nurse frustration, staff shortages, and increases in workplace violence as well as many nurses seeing the need to advocate for patient safety prompted nurses to seek ways to inform the public of their working situation. One such way was to organize or form a union. In 2020, the National Labor Relations Board (NLRB) reported a 14% increase in petitions for union representation in the health care industry (Pattani, 2021) and in 2022, greater than 30% of work stoppages that had 1,000 or more workers in the United States were done by nurses (Diaz, 2023). Caring for patients in the pandemic changed health care workers, leaving an impact and increasing their willingness to speak out (Pattani, 2021).

Mentoring and Role Modeling

Nursing mentorships are important in the development of future nurses. Hoover et al. (2020) defined *mentorship* as "a relationship between two people that has the specific purpose of one assisting the other to grow and develop and to increase their role effectiveness" (p. 2). However, not all mentorships are created equal, and not all mentorships offer what a nursing student or new nurse needs to be successful. Mentorship moves past just strengthening clinical care, when student nurses and new nurses will emulate staff nurses and mentors as role models for their future practice. Mentorship offers support to the nurse, providing them with the necessary tools to develop.

Once the graduate nurse becomes a practicing professional, a mentor can assist them in understanding the culture of nursing and of the workplace. However, the mentorship needs to be individualized; there are no one-size-fits-all for mentorships in nursing. Mentorships benefit new nurses, helping them find their way in the workplace as well as in their professional life by providing guidance and encouraging them to ask questions with no judgment. One of the important aspects of mentorships is role modeling. Role models are the link to socialization to the workplace. However, role modeling has been affected by chronic understaffing, unrelenting pressures, and constant change in both clinical and academic settings (Vinales, 2015).

It is important for a mentor to create an environment conducive to learning, welcoming, and integrating the student or the new nurse. When students feel they do not belong, they experience more stress, anxiety, depression, and lower self-esteem (Vinales, 2015). This was especially true during the pandemic when the hospital environment was challenged with nursing shortages, very sick patients, family support for patients, political upheaval that impacted patient care, and difficulty developing a welcoming environment. This had a profound effect on mentoring student nurses and new nurses, especially in rural settings where the number of qualified mentors was already limited and increased workloads restricted the opportunity for mentoring new nurses.

Pathman et al. (2022) stated that physical, emotional, and social destruction that resulted from the consequence of the COVID-19 pandemic has further marginalized low-income and racial and ethnic minority communities. It is not known how the pandemic has affected clinicians who provide care to these communities through safety-net practices, including clinicians participating in the National Health Service Corps (NHSC). In 2018 and 2019, the NHSC had thousands of clinicians under contract. At the onset of the pandemic, these clinicians recognized that they were the frontline providers for some of the most marginalized communities throughout the United States but that the NHSC service contracts did not adequately address the crises of a pandemic (Pathman et al., 2022). "The NHSC has provided support to these clinicians to reconcile pandemic related care and job changes with their contract obligations, extending contracts to accommodate periods of work-hour reductions and furloughs, and providing flexibility to allow telework and new temporary work sites" (Pathman, et al., 2022, p. 150). Pathman et al. (2022) designed a study with the aim to better understand how the COVID-19 pandemic had impacted the lives of NHSC clinicians who provided care to low-income and racial and ethnic minorities. During the later months in 2020, the researchers surveyed these clinicians serving in the NHSC in 20 states. Clinicians were asked to report on work and job changes, their personal feelings of well-being, and other lifestyle measures. Analyses were adjusted for differences in subgroup response rates and the clustering of clinicians within practice.

There were 4,263 clinicians surveyed; 1,890 (44.3%) responded. Work for the majority of health care providers was affected by the pandemic, including 64.5% whose outpatient visit numbers fell by 50% and 62.5% for whom most visits occurred virtually. A minority of clinicians experienced changes in their jobs; for example, only 14.9% had been furloughed. Three quarters (76.6%) of these NHSC clinicians scored at-risk levels for their well-being. Compared with primary care and behavioral health clinicians, dental clinicians much more often had been furloughed and had their practices closed temporarily (Pathman et al., 2022).

Findings from this research highlighted work and lifestyle disruptions that were experienced along with mental health stressors of NHSC clinicians in ways similar to its reported effects on the general population of outpatient providers. Pathman et al. (2022) recommend that mental health supports be prioritized for NHSC clinicians to minimize patient disengagement and job turnover. The research emphasizes that national programs and policies should help safety-net practices build cultures that support and give greater priority to clinicians' work, job, and mental health needs.

Conclusion

The transition to nursing and health practice for new graduates is often filled with challenges and obstacles. These factors were dramatically enhanced because of the rapid spread of the COVID-19 pandemic and the failures of government and health care leaders to proactively create strategies that may have mitigated the crises new practitioners were introduced to as they began their professional career. These issues must be examined by stakeholders at all levels of health care and be supported by federal and state legislatures and private funding sources so that we are better prepared in the future.

Questions for Discussion Related to Case Study 14.1

1. Discuss potential strategies that the nurse manager can utilize regarding issues of grief, loss, compassion fatigue, and workplace shortages to address Jacob's needs and the needs of new graduates working in rural areas.
2. How can the nurse manager mobilize her experienced staff to consider participating in a mentoring program for new graduates? Are there incentives that could be

created for experienced nurses who enjoy working with new graduates that would allow them to gain experience and professional recognition as mentors?

3. The nurse managers would like to proceed with the creation of a mentoring program and a nurse residency program. They recognize that each of these initiatives will require time, staffing, education, and financial support. What stakeholders should be mobilized to create a plan to address these opportunities?

References

Baldwin, K. M., Sleutel, M., Urban, R. W., Wells, J. N., Behan, D., Walsh, J., & Newcomb, P. (2021). An exploration of new graduate nurses' transition to specialty practice. *Journal for Nurses in Professional Development, 37*(2), 93–100. https://doi.org/10.1097/NND.0000000000000695

Buerhaus, P. I., DesRoches, C. M., Dittus, R., & Donelan, K. (2015). Practice characteristics of primary care nurse practitioners and physicians. *Nursing Outlook, 63*(2), 144–153. https://doi.org/10.1016/j.outlook.2014.08.008

Davidson, A. (2023, March 23). COVID-19 and how it's changed nursing: A two year reflection. *Nurse Journal.* https://nursejournal.org/articles/covid-19-how-its-changing-nursing/

Diaz, J. (2023, May 2). *Nearly a third of nurses nationwide say they are likely to leave the profession.* National Public Radio. npr.org/2023/05/02/1173107527/nursing-staff-crisis

Edwards, D., Hawker, C., Carrier, J., & Rees, C. (2015). A systematic review of the effectiveness of strategies and interventions to improve the transition from student to newly qualified nurse. *International Journal of Nursing Studies, 52*(7), 1254–1268. https://doi.org/10.1016/j.ijnurstu.2015.03.007

Health Resources Service Administration. (2023). *COVID-19 frequently asked questions.* https://bphc.hrsa.gov/initiatives/covid-19-information-health-centers-partners/faq

Hoover, J., Koon, A. D., Rosser, E. N., & Roa, K. D. (2020). Mentoring the working nurse: A scoping review. *Human Resources for Health, 18,* 52. https://doi.org/10.1186/s12960-020-00491-x

Meleis, A. I., Sawyer, L. M., Im, E., Hilfinger Messias, D. K., & Schumacher, K. (2010). Experiencing transitions: An emerging middle-range theory. In A. I. Meleis (Ed.), *Transitions theory: Middle range and situation specific theories in nursing research and practice* (pp. 52–84). Springer.

National Council of State Boards of Nursing. (2023). *NCLEX fact sheets.* https://www.ncsbn.org/public-files/NCLEX_Stats_2023_Q4_PassRates.pdf

Pathman, D. E., Sonis, J., Harrison, J. N., Sewell, R. G., Fannell, J., Overbeck, M., & Konrad, T. R. (2022). Experiences of safety-net practice clinicians participating in the National Health Service Corps during the COVID-19 pandemic. *Public Health Reports, 137*(1), 149–162. https://doi.org/10.1177/00333549211054083

Pattani, A. (2021, January 11). *For health care workers, the pandemic is fueling renewed interest in unions.* National Public Radio. npr.org/sections/health-shots/2021/01/11/955128562/for-health-care-workers-the-pandemic-is-fueling-renewed-intrest-in-unions

Phillips, K., Dzurec, L., Burgess, A., Beauvais, A. & McNutt-Clarke, B. (2023). Ramifications of the COVID-19 Pandemic on Nursing Students' Transition to Practice. *Journal for Nurses in Professional Development, 39* (6), E196–E201. doi: 10.1097/NND.0000000000000904.

Munn, A. C., George, T. P., Phillips, T. A., Kershner, S. H., & Hucks, J. M. (2022). Resilience and GRIT among undergraduate nursing students during the COVID 19 pandemic. *International Journal of Nursing Education Scholarship, 19*(1). https://doi.org/10.1515/ijnes-2022-0012

Roberts, S., Warren, T., & Moore, L. C. (2022). COVID-19 pandemic: Effects of replacing clinical hours with virtual simulation in BSN prelicensure nursing education. *Nursing Education Perspectives, 43*(5), 306–308. https://doi.org/10.1097/01.NEP.0000000000001002

Rural Health Information Hub. (2023). *3RNET recruitment and retention assistance.* https://www.ruralhealthinfo.org/funding/2302

Smith, S. M., Buckner, M., Jessee, M. A., Robbins, V., Horst, T., & Ivory, C. H. (2021). Impact of COVID-19 on new graduate nurses' transition to practice: Loss or gain? *Nurse Educator, 46*(4), 209–214. https://doi.org/10.1097/NNE.0000000000001042

Stellflug, S. M., Buerhaus, P., & Auerbach, D. (2022). Characteristics of family nurse practitioners and their preparation for practice in rural vs urban employment settings. *Nursing Outlook, 70*(3), 391–400. https://doi.org/10.1016/j.outlook.2021.12.007

U.S. Department of Health and Human Services, Health Resources & Services Administration. (2020, November 5). *Coronavirus (COVID-19) frequently asked questions.* National Health Service Corps and Nurse Corps. https://www.cms.gov/files/document/03092020-covid-19-faqs-508.pdf

Vinales, J. J. (2015). The mentor as a role model and the importance of belongingness. *British Journal of Nursing, 24*(10), 532–535. https://doi.org/10.12968/bjon.2015.24.10532

Wenxia, Z., Feifei, C., Min, H., Li, C., Aihong, L., & Xingfeng, L. (2022). The status and associated factors of junior nurses' transition shock: A cross-sectional study. *Journal of Nursing Management, 30*(3), 716–723. https://doi.org/10.1111/jonm.13543

UNIT VI

Continuum of Care

n the past, nurses have always been the ones who have tried to keep the patient's best interest in the forefront, to maintain empathy for what the patient and family members are experiencing. However, as staffing shortages become even greater, demands on nurses have increased, leaving little time for this empathetic and compassionate care. "There is a growing emphasis in policy, practice and research on the caring dimension of health care, in an ever-more complex context and amid financial constraints and increasing demand to meet key performance indicators, outcomes and efficiencies" (Murray & Tuqiri, 2020, p. 3).

This unit will provide insight into the impact of COVID-19 and U.S. policies affecting the care of millions of Americans. U.S. residents were challenged by public health restrictions and limited health care which lead to rapid changes in the U.S. health care system. As more and more facilities converted complete units and other nontraditional care spaces into units to treat specific COVID-19 patients, a subset of patients is left to be cared for in nontraditional fashion. However, the shortage of staff, particularly nurses, who provide patient care resulted in a change in the quality-of-care patients received during the pandemic.

Reference

Murray, S. J., & Tuqiri, K. A. (2020). The art of caring—Understanding compassionate care through storytelling. *International Practice Development Journal*, *10*(1), 1–13. https://doi.org/10.19043/ipdj.101.004

CHAPTER 15

Providing Safe and Compassionate Care in the Home Setting

"Home health services are critical to the health and social well-being of older adults, people with disabilities, and the chronically ill" (Markkanen et al., 2021, p. 2). Home care is an important alternative to facility-based care such as skilled nursing facilities (SNF) and assisted living facilities that allow individuals to stay in their home near their family and friends. In 2019, it was estimated there were 2.3 million home care workers in the United States providing services and support to assist individuals to remain safely in their homes (Tyler et al., 2021).

The home health industry has had long-standing challenges that were made worse by the pandemic. Staffing shortages worsened after the pandemic. Staff left their job due to exposure to the virus. Some older workers and people with underlying conditions that made them more susceptible to hospitalization if exposed to COVID-19 chose to leave the field or retire (Tyler et al., 2021). School and childcare closures had an impact on home health, as some staff needed to leave their positions to care for their families. For other staff, transportation presented a challenge as some felt unsafe using public transportation and people were uncomfortable having people in their homes who had been on public transportation.

The COVID-19 pandemic had an impact on home health. Some states did not recognize home care workers as "essential workers," delaying access to PPE, testing, and vaccinations (Tyler et al., 2021). This delay in recognizing home health workers as essential workers also led to difficulties accessing some clients living in residential facilities, decreasing patient volume. Most home health agencies experienced a decline in revenue due to this decline in patients.

Many home health agencies were compensated for their losses due to the federal government's response. Some agencies took advantage of the $1.7 billion from the U.S. Centers for Medicare and Medicaid Services, while other agencies were able to receive funding through the Provider Relief Fund (Holly, 2020). In addition, all Medicare-certified home health agencies benefited from Congress's decision to suspend the 2% Medicare appropriation (Holly, 2020).

While there was an overall decrease in the number of patients referred to home health agencies, there was an increase (5%–6%) in the number of Medicare non-COVID-19 patients referred to home health agencies during the pandemic (Koenig et al., 2022). This shift is likely due to the concerns the patient and their provider had related to the risk of a COVID-19 infection (Koenig et al., 2022). Receiving treatment at home reduced some of the concerns related to contracting COVID; however, home health clients were still impacted. When interviewed, clients identified five themes (Markkanen et al., 2021):

- fear of risk of infection, which led to clients being worried about contracting the virus, suspending home care services for a time
- less physical connection with others, leading to decreases in client–caregiver communication
- little change prior to the pandemic related to caregivers performing the same duties
- telehealth use, which was limited, and phone use being the most common use of communication for case managers and providers
- wearing masks, limiting the ability to see facial expressions and to read lips

Home health agency managers in Massachusetts who were surveyed during the month of June 2020 identified the COVID-19 impact on agencies, clients, and aides (Sama et al., 2021). Eighty percent of the respondents reported a decrease in the number of home health aide visit hours per client hours. The decreases were related to patient preference and COVID-19 policies (Betsy Lehman Center for Patient Safety, 2020). Ninety-nine percent of the clients were unwilling to have a home health aide in their home, reporting that their family members can complete the roles of the aide (64%). In addition, home health aides were unwilling to go into client's homes (74%) for fear of being exposed to the virus. Due to COVID-19 policies and nationwide shutdowns, many aides were not available as they needed to care for their children and family members (74%; Figure 15.1).

81% OF AGENCIES REPORTED A DECREASE IN HOME CARE HOURS

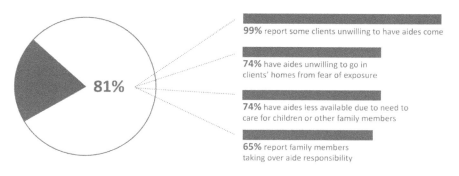

FIGURE 15.1 Causes of decrease in home care hours.

Challenges to Home Health Settings

Before the pandemic, there was a shifting of patients from skilled nursing facilities (SNF) to home health agencies. For 2 decades before the pandemic there was an increase in patients who were referred to home health agencies over skilled nursing facilities. The first shift was noted in 2009 when the SNF days for Medicare beneficiaries decreased by 15% from 1,808 to 1,539 (Holly, 2020). This change was initiated in part by referral from in-patient hospital discharges. In the first quarter of 2019, 23.3% of hospital discharges were referred to home health versus 21.1% who were referred to SNF (Holly, 2020; Figure 15.2). Some of these changes can be related to the number of deaths among long-term care residents and workers. *USA Today* reported that more than 40,6000 long-term residents and workers died because of COVID-19, approximately 40% of the U.S.'s overall death rate (Holly, 2020). Due to these statistics, it is not surprising that over 50% of family members are more likely to choose in-home care for a family member than they would have prior to the pandemic (Holly, 2020).

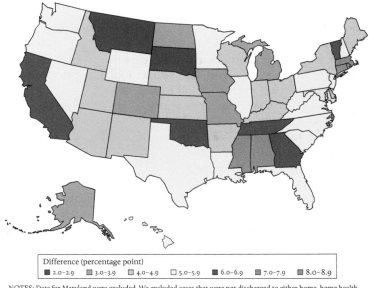

NOTES: Data for Maryland were excluded. We excluded cases that were not discharged to either home, home health, skilled nursing, facility, inpatient rehabilitation facility, or long-term care hospital.

Data: KNG Health analysis of 2017–2021 Medicare claims data.

FIGURE 15.2 Changes in state-level rates of hospital discharge to home health agencies from prepandemic to pandemic periods.

Some of the challenges home health agencies faced were addressed by changes to policies, regulations, and guidance from state and federal agencies. Some states accessed funds from the CARES Act or other state funding to provide increased Medicaid payment rates to home health agencies (Figure 15.3) to purchase PPE and distribute bonuses, hazard pay, and retainers for staff.

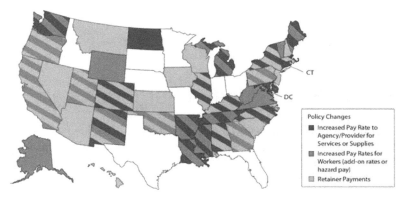

FIGURE 15.3 States that made policy changes to increase Medicaid payment rates.

Home health agencies had already been moving toward the use of telehealth before the pandemic. With the demand of social distancing, telehealth became a viable method of monitoring patients. In April 2019, then President Trump indicated that the number of patients using telehealth increased from about 11,000 to more than 650,000 a week (Holly, 2020). This demonstrated the expansion and value of telehealth. The CARES Act also encouraged the use of telehealth. However, while agencies were using telehealth to access their patients, they were unable to be reimbursed through Medicare.

Policy changes at the federal and state level shifted training and employment requirements allowing for the use of telehealth (Tyler et al., 2021). Thirty-two states made changes to pre-employment requirements to address the staffing shortage. These changes allowed staff to be trained virtually or delay certain pre-employment requirements (Figure 15.4).

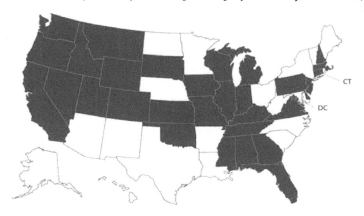

FIGURE 15.4 State policy changes related to employment requirements and qualifications.

Changes in state and federal policies also lead to new and increased pay for family caregivers, who were paid to care for family members in 34 states. During the pandemic, many individuals worked from home, giving them the opportunity to care for their family members while decreasing out-of-pocket costs (Figure 15.5).

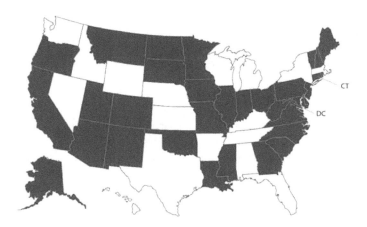

FIGURE 15.5 State policy changes allowing payment of increased payment to family caregivers.

Positive Changes

While there have been challenges for home health agencies during the pandemic, there have been positive changes. The pandemic has been the catalyst for home health agencies to adapt their services with new technologies and enhance infection-prevention measures (Mills, 2022). The demand for home health is expected to grow in the next decade as almost 70% of Americans will be turning 65 years of age and may need support in the future (Mills, 2022). During the pandemic clients utilizing home health services were concerned about contracting COVID. However, patients are more at risk of contracting COVID in an acute care setting, making home health care a safe alternative.

Home health agencies changed policies and practices to address the challenges resulting from the pandemic. The ability for nonphysician practitioners to order home health and home care services was a positive result. This contributed to an increase in the number of clients, reversing the losses that occurred at the beginning of the pandemic. Infection-control practices also changed during the pandemic as agencies focused heavily on infection control and access to PPE to maintain in-person care. Shifting to new virtual processes by adding telehealth services to continue to provide care and monitor clients remotely allowed for patients to be monitored in their home with decreased risk of infection. These services ranged from medication reminders to conducting physical therapy sessions using videoconferencing.

Conclusion

Most stakeholders have outlined changes that need to occur in home health in the future. The following ongoing challenges could be addressed to improve the situation for home care (Tyler et al., 2021):

- ensuring that homecare workers are designated as essential workers
- providing home health employees with priority access to PPE, testing, and vaccines
- improving wages of home health employees, especially aides, personal care workers, and direct service providers, to improve retention
- improving career opportunities for workers by offering better training and career advancement
- standardizing training and other requirements across all states to make these more transferrable
- providing government reimbursement for certain telehealth services

While many stakeholders see the need for continued change, they do hope for increased availability of home- and community-based services and increased appreciation of home-care workers for the essential role they play in keeping clients safe in their homes and communities. The U.S. homecare market increased from 2017 to 2020, with projections that the market will continue to rise from 2021 to 2025. This increase is due to an aging population, increasing prevalence of chronic diseases, and increasing per-capita personal income in a low-cost setting.

Kathy is a registered nurse who has been working for a rural home care agency as a certified wound care nurse for more than 20 years. This morning Kathy is scheduled to see James Loury, a 62-year-old patient who was discharged from an urban hospital nearly 100 miles from his home. His hospitalization was the result of the trauma he sustained when he attempted to repair his faulty car engine. James sustained second-degree burns on his right calf, right thigh, and the lower portion of his right abdomen. While hospitalized, James underwent debridement of his burns, antibiotic therapy, and skin grafts to his right thigh.

As Kathy traveled the rural route to James's house, she noticed that her cell phone signal had been lost. She was not surprised since she had seen patients in this area before. When she pulled into James's lot, she noticed multiple vehicles that looked in need of repair. There was no doorbell to ring, so she knocked on the door and said, "Hi Mr. Loury, I'm Kathy, the nurse from homecare. She heard a voice from the back of the house say, "Come in." Upon entering the living room, she saw James entering with a walker from the kitchen. James stood 6 feet, 4 inches tall. She also noticed several guns hanging over the mantel and a large pocketknife on the table. She felt a bit on edge but reminded herself that James needed her care and expertise.

1. What are the risks to the nurse in this situation? Are there alternative options for care given these risks?
2. What are the risks to this patient if Kathy refuses to provide care?
3. Does the homecare agency have an obligation to put measures in place to maximize safety for nurses who provide care for rural and remote residents?
4. Identify the community stakeholders who should be involved in advocacy initiatives to address these concerns.

References

Betsy Lehman Center for Patient Safety. (2020). *The impact of COVID-19 on home health and home care in Massachusetts*. UMass Lowell Safe Home Care Project.

Holly, R. (2020). *Predicting COVID-19's long-term impact on the home health care market*. Home Health Care News. https://homehealthcarenews.com/2020/06/predicting-covid-19s-long-term-impact-on-the-home-health-care-market/

Koenig, L., Steele-Adjognon, M., Hamlett, E., Cintina, I., & Unuigbe, A. (2022, July 14). *Did COVID-19 have a disparate impact on home health use in Medicare?* The Commonwealth Fund. https://www.commonwealthfund.org/publications/issue-briefs/2022/jul/did-covid-19-have-disparate-impact-home-health-use-medicare

Markkanen, P., Brouillette, N., Quinn, M., Galligan, C., Sama, S., Lindberg, J., & Karlsson, N. (2021). "It changed everything": The safe home care qualitative study of the COVID-19 pandemic's impact on home care aides, clients, and managers. *BMC Health Services Research, 21*(1), 1055.

Mills, S. (2022, January 19). *Homecare: How COVID-19 reinforced the important role of home health care.* Cahaba Media Group. https://www.homecaremag.com/january-2022/how-covid-19-reinforced-role-home-health

Sama, S. R., Quinn, M. M., Galligan, C. J., Karlsson, N. D., Gore, R. J., Kriebel, D., Prentice, J. C., Osei-Poku, G., Carter, C. N., Markkanen, P. K., & Lindberg, J. E. (2021). Impacts of the COVID-19 pandemic on home health and home care agency managers, clients, and aides: A cross-sectional survey, March to June, 2020. *Home Health Care Management & Practice, 33*(2), 125–129. https://doi.org/10.1177/1084822320980415

Tyler, D., Hunter, M., Mulmule, N., & Porter, K. (2021). *COVID-19 intensifies home care workforce challenges: Policy perspectives issue brief.* Office of the Assistant Secretary for Planning and Evaluation, U.S. Department of Health and Human Services. https://aspe.hhs.gov/reports/covid-19-intensifies-home-care-workforce-challenges-policy-perspectives-issue-brief

Image Credits

CHAPTER 16

The Impact of COVID-19 on Nurses Providing Palliative and Hospice Care

The COVID-19 pandemic has brought about many unforeseen challenges for rural nurses providing palliative and hospice care. The elimination of visitations for end-of-life patients posed unique barriers in rural areas where geographic distance and poor telecommunication services often add to the isolation of these patients and loved ones. Jeitziner et al. (2021) stated that nurses in rural areas continue to be particularly creative in establishing connections for families and patients during their final weeks and days in order to lessen the complicated grief and symptoms of PTSD. This chapter details the lived experiences of nurses on the frontlines of both inpatient and community settings who struggled to provide compassionate end-of-life care while allowing loved ones to effectively process their grief and loss during the COVID-19 pandemic.

The National Institute on Aging (NIA) defines *palliative care* as a unique care model for persons of any age with serious illnesses, such as cancer or heart failure. These patients may receive medical care for their symptom management, palliative care, and treatments aimed at curing their serious illnesses. There are distinct and subtle differences between palliative and hospice care (NIA, 2021). Hospice care focuses on the physical care and comfort of persons with serious illnesses at the end of life. Hospice supports individuals and their care providers with interventions when the person's illness does not respond to medical attempts to cure it or slow the progression of the disease (NIA, 2021). If an individual can no longer make their own health care decisions, a caregiver or family member may have to take on those responsibilities.

Palliative care can effectively address the distressing physical, emotional, psychological, and spiritual suffering related to either serious acute or chronic conditions; additionally, it can be delivered at the same time as usual treatment at any point in the disease trajectory to improve the quality of life for those individuals living in rural and remote areas (Tasseff et al., 2019). Often, persons receiving palliative care will transition into a hospice model of care at the end of life. However, a significant gap exists in the research pertaining to the access and impact of palliative and hospice care in rural and remote areas.

Palliative Care: A Basic Human Right

The WHO (2020) sees palliative care as a basic human right. However, a mere 14% of persons globally who qualify for palliative care actually take advantage of the physical, psychological, and spiritual support that this specialized care can offer to patients and their families. Basic palliative care interventions, such as proper positioning, massage, and environmental changes, can typically be delivered by family or friends. More complex interventions such as medication modifications, changes in prescribed treatment regimens, and other forms of palliative medicine require the oversight of trained palliative care providers. Tasseff et al. (2019) state that middle-range palliative care strategies can be simultaneously implemented as a component of comprehensive primary care across rural areas. This caring approach can offer residents in rural communities the opportunity to remain active for longer periods of time, with an optimal quality of life while, ideally, aging in place.

The Hospice Experience Outside of the United States: The Canadian Perspective

There is a gap in the literature regarding hospice experiences in the rural United States, but reviewing the unique option that exists for patients with terminal illnesses in Canada to end their suffering with medically assisted suicide can offer some insight. In 2016, the Supreme Court in Canada legalized medically assisted suicide. The Court also declared that no health care provider can be required to provide medical assistance in dying. The Canadian Nurses Association (2023), in congruence with other guidelines for health care professionals across the globe, supports the nurse's right to opt out of participation in medical assistance in dying. A team of researchers recognized that some nurses declared a conscientious objection to this type of care, resulting in the potential for a lack of availability of nurses who will provide this care in rural settings: "Exercising conscientious objection to medical assistance in dying in rural and remote areas, by way of policies developed with an urban focus, is one example of how the needs of rural nurses and their rural patients may not be met, leading to issues of patient access to medical assistance in dying and retention of nursing staff" (Panchuk & Thirsk, 2021, p. 766). The researchers illustrate the multifaceted concerns of the conscientious objection of nurses to medical assistance in dying and the retention of nursing staff in these settings.

Due to various physical, emotional, and social constraints, rural and remote environments may add to the challenges that nurses must address to act congruently with their ethics when making decisions about patients and care plans, including the overlap in roles that rural nurses must balance as family members, neighbors, parishioners, and nurses within their communities. Additionally, it is important to consider that these nurses may face conflicts surrounding power dynamics with providers or leaders and concerns surrounding retaliation because of their conscientious objection to medically assisted dying. Panchuk and Thirsk (2021) adapted an ethical decision-making framework from MacDonald's (2010) framework to provide step-by-step guidance using reflective questioning, with the aim of thorough and thoughtful patient-centered decision-making principles. Table 16.1 outlines the six steps that provide a foundation that, if applied thoughtfully and carefully, brings a deeper understanding of the phenomenon of conscientious objection. MacDonald (2010) states that these steps do not have to be completed in a particular order.

TABLE 16.1 A Guide to Moral Decision-Making

Recognizing the moral decision	Remember that important clues include conflicts between two or more values or ideals.
Who are the interested parties? What are their relationships?	Carefully identify stakeholders in the decision. Be imaginative and sympathetic. Consider that there are more parties whose interests should be taken into consideration than is immediately obvious.
What values or principles are involved?	Think through the shared values that are at stake in making this decision. Is there a question of trust? Is personal autonomy a consideration? Is there a question of fairness? Is anyone to be harmed or helped?
Weigh the benefits and the burdens.	Benefits—broadly defined—might include such things as the production of goods (physical, emotional, financial, social, etc.) for various parties, the satisfaction of preferences, and acting in accordance with various relevant values (e.g., fairness). Burdens might include causing physical or emotional pain to various parties, imposing financial costs, and ignoring relevant values.
Look for analogous cases.	Can you think of other similar decisions? What course of action was taken? Was it a good decision? How is the present case like that one? How is it different?
Discuss with relevant others.	The merits of discussion should not be underestimated. Time permitting, discuss your decision with as many people who have a stake in it. Gather opinions and ask for the reasons behind those opinions. Remember that your ability to discuss with others may be limited by expectations and rules about confidentiality.

Source: Chris MacDonald, Selections from "A Guide to Moral Decision Making," http://www.ethicsweb.ca/ guide/guide2010.pdf. Copyright © 2010 by Chris MacDonald. Reprinted with permission.

Comparing the Quality of Hospice Care Between Rural and Urban Community Residents

Baernholdt et al. (2015) identified multiple challenges to delivering hospice care in rural areas. Those challenges include geography, weather, resources, hospice staff shortages, and the characteristics and culture of the residents within rural communities. The research team sought to examine whether perceptions of the quality of hospice care and if that quality differed in rural and urban communities and between patients and families. The study was supported by the quality health outcomes model (QHOM). The QHOM is based on Donabedian's model, which has been a foundational model for evaluating and comparing health care quality for more than 60 years. The Donabedian model of quality underscores the synergistic relationships between structure, process, and outcomes (Huseman-Maratea et al., 2022). The QHOM was adapted for the study to evaluate the quality of hospice care by linking hospice interventions to patient/family outcomes through the system or patient characteristics (Baernholdt et al., 2015). The study addressed specific hospice interventions that are associated with hospice outcomes in rural and urban regions.

The system characteristics were measured as geographic and care locations. This information was obtained from admission data. Geographic location was identified as rural or urban using the patients' residential ZIP code, and the county codes from the CDC were obtained. The researchers then merged the county codes with the Economic Research Service's rural/urban continuum codes to determine whether the care was delivered in a rural or urban location (Baernholdt et al., 2015). Care locations were described as either at-home or inpatient hospice settings. There were three variables used to define patient characteristics; race/ethnicity was White, African American, or other. The primary diagnosis was classified as cancer or noncancer. The person who answered the survey questions described their relationship to the patient as self, spouse, adult child, or other.

Hospice interventions included three binary variables: an explanation of the care plan, information about the patient's condition, and emotional support. Each of these was measured as whether an intervention had been provided. Hospice outcomes included overall satisfaction, satisfaction with pain management, and satisfaction with symptom management. Each of these variables measured whether the person was satisfied with the hospice care (Baernholdt et al., 2015).

Study Findings

Results from the Baernholdt et al. study (2015) show a total of 743 (331 rural and 412 urban) surveys were included. During the data collection period, 2,073 patients were admitted to the hospice, but 621 died before being surveyed, 617 patients could not be reached or did not want to participate, and 92 surveys were duplicates (n = 242) or had missing data (n = 68). Overall, satisfaction, satisfaction with pain management, and satisfaction with other symptom management received positive ratings (Baernholdt et al., 2015). For overall satisfaction, only three rural patients were not satisfied.

Data analysis using multivariate logistic regression showed the outcome satisfaction with pain management; only the intervention explanation of the care plan was not significant; whether the patient or others were surveyed was not significant. For the two hospice outcomes, the rural location was approaching significance (pain management odds ratio = 1.54; p =.19; symptom management odds ratio = 1.97; p = .06). Although the outcome, overall satisfaction did not meet the assumption of more than five cases per cell when logical regression was performed; all three care interventions were significant, as was the rural location (Baernholdt et al., 2015). The researchers emphasize that these findings provide evidence for the need for hospice providers to ensure that they incorporate all three interventions: explanation of plan of care, information about the patient's condition, and emotional support to provide the highest level of care satisfaction.

Exploring the Perceptions of Rural Dwellers Regarding Palliative Care

Tasseff et al. (2017) conducted a qualitative study to understand the perception of rural-dwelling veterans regarding palliative care. The researchers recruited six rural veterans in a geographic area that included more than 8,500 square miles. Rural nursing theory provided the conceptual framework for the study. Audio recorded, semi-structured in-person interviews were scheduled with the participants, and the researchers used an interview guide as the foundation for each interview. The characteristics of the study participants are summarized in Table 16.2.

TABLE 16.2 Rural Veterans-Participant Characteristics

Demographics	Veterans n (%)
Males	6 (100)
Marital Status	
Married	5 (83.3)
Divorced	1 (16.7)
Race	
White	6 (100)
Education	
HS grad/GED	2 (33.3)
Some college	1 (16.7)
Associate's	1 (16.7)
Bachelor's	2 (33.3)
Employment	
< 35 hours	3 (50.0)
Not employed	3 (50.0)
Veteran Status[a]	
Noncombat	4 (66.7)
Combat	2 (33.3)
Military retiree	1 (16.7)
Branch of Service	
Air Force	3 (50)
Army	2 (33.3)
Navy	1 (16.7)
Era	
Vietnam	5 (83.3)
Desert Storm, OEF, OIF[b]	1 (16.7)
Service-connected disability: Yes	3 (50.0)
Disability rating	
30%	1 (33.3)
70%	1 (33.3)
100%	1 (33.3)
Age (Years)	66.8 (8.0)
Length of Service (Years)	7.9 (7.1)
Rural (Years)[c]	57.4 (26.9)
Current (Years)[d]	21.1 (22.7)

Note: (a) Total years, over an entire life, living rurally; (b) Operation Enduring Freedom, Operation Iraqi Freedom; (c) total years of living rurally, over a lifetime; (d) total years lived in the area of current ZIP code (postal code).

Source: Tasseff et al. (2019).

Data Collection

A member of the research team who was a resident in the study area conducted each participant interview. Before the larger data collection began, a pilot interview was conducted with a rural veteran using the semi-structured research guide. The results of the pilot interview were not included in the final data collection. The following questions were asked during each of the interviews:

- How would you define palliative care, or what is your personal definition of palliative care?
- Where is palliative care delivered?
- When is the most appropriate time for palliative care?

Additional demographic data were collected using a short questionnaire that included gender, marital status, ethnicity, race, birth year, ZIP code of home and work, total years of rural living, years lived in current ZIP code, level of education, and employment. Hand-written field notes and memos were created following the interviews.

Emerging Themes

Four themes were illuminated from these interviews: a lack of understanding and uncertainty regarding palliative care; where and when; palliative care not as hospice care; and opportunities. The study participants lacked awareness of the meaning of palliative care. Five of the six participants did not perceive palliative care to be end of life. However, none of the participants perceived palliative care to be hospice care.

Findings

Although these rural veteran participants were unable to define palliative care and were uncertain about its meaning, all of them were able to describe chronic illnesses that lasted for decades (Tasseff et al., 2019). Each rural veteran was familiar with hospice care, although they did not relate palliative care with hospice care. Five of the six veterans did not perceive palliative care to be end-of-life care. Similar to the findings of McIlfatrick et al. (2014) and Golla et al. (2014), a lack of understanding about palliative care was found among these rural veterans. Tasseff et al. (2019) emphasizes that nurses caring for veterans in rural areas must enhance their skills as change agents and advocates to provide a good life and death for our nation's veterans.

Pediatric Hospice Care in Rural Regions

Weaver (2018) detailed the challenges she witnessed upon returning to her supportive oncology practice in rural Nebraska. Her caseload of patients frequently included those who needed to travel about 4 hours to the closest pediatric hospital and more than 1 hour to the closest adult health care facility. "After using our state-wide hospice service database and an internet search to locate hospice services for a terminally ill child and her family, neither of the rural hospices felt they were able to provide home hospice services which would have allowed the child and her family to spend her last days at home with care" (Weaver, 2018, p. 517). The child was referred to a family practice physician who rotated at the elder care hospice facility, which was located 40 minutes from the patient's home. The provider became this child's primary hospice physician with ongoing consultation from the pediatric hospice team. The nurse at the child's elementary school and the school counselor were notified of the plan to bring the patient home, and they offered to join the support team for the child and the family. Although the pediatric oncologist was concerned that the growing care team would be too overwhelming for the family, they welcomed the additional members to the team and said they were comforted by their familiarity (Weaver, 2018). The parents also asked that their daughter's youth minister continue to serve as her spiritual support while she was receiving hospice care since he had baptized her in the prior year. The hospice chaplain agreed and offered to mentor the family's pastor in grief and bereavement topics, and a strong bond was formed with the common goal of supporting the family unit through their hospice journey and beyond (Weaver, 2018).

The pediatric oncologist continued her 4-hour commute to visit the patient and her family on Saturdays for several weeks. She learned the importance of closeness from this family and recalled finding sleeping bags beside the patient's bed for her three siblings and parents. They spent time each evening telling stories about the patient's lessons and how being a part of her family helped them grow closer to their faith (Weaver, 2018).

This patient's story is filled with challenges and opportunities that are unique to hospice care in rural areas. Nurses and health care professionals must advocate for funding to create medical homes in these regions to keep families close to their roots and their health care providers as they navigate toward their end of life, regardless of their age or circumstances.

CASE STUDY 16.1

The Gove family relocated to a rural town in the northwestern United States in 2018. Ted was passionate about his job as an environmental engineer for a large construction company that promoted green construction. Kyra was a registered nurse who worked for a critical access hospital (CAH). The couple had two children, Evan who was 9 years old, and Mya who was 16 months old. Evan had been diagnosed with type I neurofibromatosis at the age of 4, and he experienced multiple hospitalizations throughout his childhood. The family had hoped that the move to the northwest would offer a more holistic environment for Evan despite the 90-mile distance from the Gove's home to the urban medical center where Evan's doctors practiced. Both Ted and Kyra had become active members of their local church and often volunteered their time and resources.

In January 2020 Evan experienced sudden vision loss, and he was diagnosed with an inoperable intracranial glioma. The neurologist and neuro-oncologist referred Evan and his family to palliative care services, understanding that he may transition to hospice services in a matter of months. Kyra began to research hospice services in the area, and she became incredibly concerned about the lack of available services to meet the needs of pediatric hospice patients and their families.

In early February 2020, Kyra expressed these concerns during a virtual visit with Amy, a nurse practitioner from the neuro-oncology service, and the nurse agreed to help her "imagine" Evan's care team. One week later, Amy was able to connect with a neurologist whose practice was located 35 miles from the Gove's home. The neurologist's specialty was primarily geriatric neurology. He spent the majority of his time conducting dementia screenings at a local community clinic. However, he understood the challenges of finding pediatric hospice specialists, and he offered to be the primary provider if Amy would continue on as a member of Evan's care team.

The Impact of Telehealth on Palliative and Hospice Care Delivery in Rural Areas

There is a gap in the literature regarding the effects of telehealth and remote patient monitoring in persons needing palliative care in rural communities. Bonsignore et al. (2018) initiated a research study with the following objectives: "Describe a telehealth palliative care program using the TapCloud remote patient monitoring application and videoconferencing; evaluate the feasibility of, usability, and acceptability of a telehealth system in palliative care; and use a quality data assessment collection tool in addition to TapCloud ratings of symptom burden and hospice transitions" (p. 7).

The researchers designed a mixed-methods approach to assess the practicality, usefulness, and acceptability of a system designed specifically to support palliative care patients. Quantitative data were collected on patient symptom burden and improvement, hospice transitions, and advance directives (Bonsignore et al., 2018). Semi-structured interviews were conducted with a subpopulation of telehealth patients, family members, caregivers, and health care providers to better understand their experiences using TapCloud.

Findings from this study highlight the feasibility and acceptability of this telehealth model for a rural population of patients in Western North Carolina (Bonsignore et al., 2018). Typically, this type of rural area faces health care disparities daily due to a lack of access to care for patients with emergent needs. However, because the researchers were able to capture real-time patient symptom data, the TapCloud alerts sent information to providers that allowed them to prevent unnecessary suffering and potential emergency room visits or hospitalizations (Bonsignore et al., 2018). The Quality Data Assessment Collection Tool (QDACT; Table 16.3) demonstrated a reduction in symptom burden, documentation of advanced directives, and a high hospice transition rate.

TABLE 16.3 Patient Symptom Burden and Symptom Improvement

Total Patients = 73	0–3	4–6	7–10	Unable to Respond	Unknown	Improvement
Pain n (%)	49 (67.1)	11 (15.1)	6 (8.2)	2 (2.7)	5 (6.9)	9/11 (81.8)
Dyspnea n (%)	57 (78.1)	9 (12.3)	2 (2.7)	1 (1.4)	4 (5.5)	7/9 (77.8)
Constipation n (%)	65 (89)	4 (5.5)	0 (0)	1 (1.4)	3 (4.1)	2/2 (100)
Tiredness n (%)	59 (80.8)	2 (2.8)	3 (4.1)	2 (2.7)	7 (9.6)	5/5 (100)
Nausea n (%)	62 (84.9)	3 (4.1)	2 (2.7)	2 (2.7)	4 (5.5)	3/4 (75)
Depression n (%)	55 (75.3)	6 (8.2)	3 (4.1)	2 (2.7)	7 (9.6)	9/10 (90)
Anxiety n (%)	59 (80.8)	3 (4.1)	4 (5.5)	2 (2.7)	5 (6.9)	2/5 (40)
Drowsiness n (%)	60 (82.3)	3. (4.1)	2 (2.7)	2 (2.7)	6 (8.2)	3/3 (100)
Appetite n (%)	55 (75.3)	5 (6.9)	3 (4.1)	2 (2.7)	8 (11)	5/9 (55.6)
Well-Being n (%)	46 (63)	15 (20.6)	2 (2.7)	4 (5.5)	6 (8.2)	11/14 (78.8)

Note: Edmonton Symptom Assessment Scale (ESAS) scores of patients using the quality data assessment collection tool (QDACT) scores at the first in-person palliative care visit. Improvement is defined as patients with a score of 4 on the first visit who have had one-point reduction in that assessment by the second or third in-person visit.

Source: Bonsignore et al. (2018).

Conclusion

Three essential elements must be in place in order for rural patients to receive the highest quality of palliative and hospice care, either in their homes or in a hospice environment. Those elements include a health care provider who is not only willing to provide care but skilled at bringing together a collaborative team to meet the needs of the patient and the family as their condition changes; a patient-centered plan of care that includes cultural competence and an ability to meet that family unit where they are in the palliative care or hospice process; and emotional support for the patient, their caregivers, and the skilled staff who may include neighbors, friends, or members of a local church community who often provide ongoing support in rural and remote areas. Future research must examine various care models based on hospice interventions and the challenges of living in a rural or remote area that must be faced when providing this specialized care.

Questions for Discussion Related to Case Study 16.1

1. Evan and his family will need a team in order to meet his care needs as his condition continues to decline. Who should comprise that team? What strategies can Amy and his physician provider utilize to identify and enlist other specialists to meet Evan's needs and the needs of his family?
2. Consider the following challenges that must be addressed in order to meet Evan's needs and propose potential strategies that would capitalize on the values of rural residents to meet those needs:
    a. *Access to prescribed medications*. How can the community help Evan and his family with the cost and transport of needed medications?
    b. *Respite care*. How can Amy assist Kyra with the coordination of respite care for Evan and childcare for Mya?
    c. *Work responsibilities*. The family has always been a two-income family. How can Kyra's work community be mobilized to provide childcare and respite so that Kyra can continue to work in a reduced or per-diem capacity? Are there current programs/services to assist both Kyra and Ted maintain their employment while prioritizing their family needs?
    d. *Support from the faith community*. How can members of the Goves' church community provide comfort, support, and services for the family?

References

Baernholdt, M., Campbell, C. L. Hinton, I. D., Yan, G., & Lewis, E. (2015). Quality of hospice care. *Journal of Nursing Care Quality*, 30(3), 247–253. https://doi.org/10.1097/NCQ.0000000000000108

Bonsignore, L., Bloom, N., Steinhauser, K., Nichols, R., Allen, T., Twaddle, M., & Bull, J. (2018). Evaluating the feasibility and acceptability of a telehealth program in a rural palliative care population: TapCloud for palliative care. *Journal of Pain and Symptom Management*, 56(1), 7–14. https://doi.org/10.1016/j.jpainsymman.2018.03.013

Canadian Nurses Association. (2023). *Medical assistance in dying.* https://www.cna-aiic.ca/en/policy-advocacy/advocacy-priorities/medical-assistance-in-dying#:~:text=Medical%20 assistance%20in%20dying%20(MAID,who%20have%20explicitly%20requested%20MAID.

Golla, H., Galushko, M., Pfaff, H., & Voltz, R. (2014). Multiple sclerosis and palliative care perceptions of severely affected multiple sclerosis patients and their health professionals: A qualitative study. *BMC Palliative Care*, *13*(1), 1–23. https://doi.org/10.1186/1472-684X-13-11

Huseman-Maratea, D., Hahn, J., Williams, E., & Morton, D. E. (2022). Application of the Donabedian model to guide Virtual Magnet® site visit preparations during a pandemic. *Nurse Leader*, *20*(6), 580–584. https://doi.org/10.1016/j.mnl.2022.03.004

Jeitziner, M.-M., Camenisch, S. A., Jenni-Moser, B., Schefold, J. C., & Zante, B. (2021). End-of-life care during the COVID-19 pandemic—What makes the difference? *Nursing in Critical Care*, *26*(3), 212–214. https://doi.org/10.1111/nicc.12593

MacDonald, C. (2010, September 25). *A guide to moral decision-making.* http://www.ethicsweb.ca/guide/guide2010.pdf

McIlfatrick, S., Noble, H., McCorry, N. K., Roulston, A., Hasson, F., McLaughlin, D., Johnston, G., Rutherford, L., Payne, C., Kernohan, G., Kelly, S., & Craig, A. (2014). Exploring public awareness and perceptions of palliative care: A qualitative study. *Palliative Medicine*, *28*(3), 273–280. https://doi.org/10.1177/0269216313502372

National Institute on Aging. (2021). *What are palliative care and hospice care?* https://www.nia.nih.gov/health/what-are-palliative-care-and-hospice-care

Panchuk, J., & Thirsk, L. M. (2021). Conscientious objection to medical assistance in dying in rural/remote nursing. *Nursing Ethics*, *28*(5), 766–775. https://doi.org/10.1177/0969733020976185

Tasseff, T. L., Tavernier, S. S., Neill, K. S., & Watkins, P. R. (2019). Exploring perceptions of palliative care among rural dwelling veterans. *Online Journal of Rural Nursing and Health Care*, *19*(1), 159–178. https://doi.org/10.14574/ojrnhc.v19i1.528

Weaver, M. S. (2018). Growing symbiotic local partnerships to nurture quality pediatric hospice care in rural regions: Companion planting. *Archives of Pediatrics & Adolescent Medicine*, *172*(6), 517–518. R https://doi.org/10.1001/jamapediatrics.2017.3910

World Health Organization. (2020, August 5). *Palliative care.* http://www.who.int/mediacentre/factsheets/fs402/en/

UNIT VII

The Future of Nursing and Lessons Learned

The COVID-19 pandemic was a challenging time for the nation and for the world. With these challenges, there is an opportunity to learn and grow, to examine those ideas that worked well and those that did not. This text has tried to present a nonjudgmental reflection of how the pandemic influenced many aspects of health care and the professionals who experienced it in many different areas and settings. However, what did we learn from the pandemic, and what changes do we need to make for future health care crises? "Novel, collaborative partnerships between schools of nursing and healthcare organizations are needed to ensure the nation is producing an adequate supply of new nurses to offset the pending nursing workforce shortage" (Michel et al., 2021, p. 911).

Health care administrators must continue to look for ways to recruit and retain staff, especially in rural settings where shortages are even more acute. Community leaders must also offer solutions that augment recruitment strategies. The nation learned that we do not live in silos anymore, that many ideas from many team members have value.

Reference

Michel, A., Ryan, N., Mattheus, D., Knopf, A., Abuelezam, N. N., Stamp, K., Branson, S., Hekel, B., & Fontenot, H. B. (2021). Undergraduate nursing students' perceptions on nursing education during the 2020 COVID-19 pandemic: A national sample. *Nursing Outlook*, *69*(5), 903–912. https://doi.org/10.1016/j.outlook.2021.05.004

CHAPTER 17

Summation

Data from the World Population Review (2023) reveals the average U.S. population density is 93.29 people per square mile. The population density of individual states has a wide range, from 1.28 people per square mile to 11,685.51 people per square mile. Most states have rural areas, including New Jersey, which is the most densely populated state with 1,259 residents per square mile. The five least densely populated states include South Dakota (11.78 residents per square mile), North Dakota (11.79 residents per square mile), Montana (7.42 residents per square mile), Wyoming (6 residents per square mile), and Alaska (1.28 residents per square mile; World Population Review, 2023).

Residents of these areas must navigate the challenges of living in rural settings that include geographic obstacles, poor or no internet connectivity, social isolation, and lack of access to health care services daily. The COVID-19 pandemic enhanced these challenges, thus compounding the daily burdens of rural residents, which were overshadowed by fears of a virus that brought government shutdowns, severe illness, death, and misinformation. All these factors contributed to widening health disparities compared to their urban counterparts.

There is growing evidence of epidemiological inequalities in the disease burden of the COVID-19 virus between urban and rural areas. Across the United States, there was minimal preparedness for the COVID-19 pandemic; however, rural areas were even less prepared due to the lack of a stable health care structure to address the acute and chronic needs of rural residents, health literacy limitations, and the vulnerability of rural residents who are aging with multiple comorbidities (Lakhani et al., 2020). This text sought to present a national picture of the lived experiences of rural frontline nurses and health care providers who faced these challenges while providing care for residents and managing the daily crises that occurred during the height of the COVID-19 pandemic.

In health care, we use debriefing to teach health care providers to examine situations to determine what improvements need to be made. "Debriefing is a direct, intentional conversation that can be used for knowledge ... to answer questions about threats to patient safety and patient care" (Edwards et al., 2021, p. 1). Debriefing is an important strategy for learning about and making improvements, but did debriefing take place during and after the COVID-19 pandemic? Did debriefing take place after the 1918 pandemic? What did we learn from the 1918 pandemic that was useful in the 2020 COVID-19 pandemic? In this text, we have discussed various areas of rural health care that were impacted by the pandemic, including some changes in health care that led to improvements and others that made access to health care for rural America more difficult.

Telehealth

In many areas of health care, the use of telehealth was in its infancy at the beginning of the pandemic. However, the limitations that were placed on patients and providers during the pandemic resulted in an increase in the use of telehealth, which offered a good alternative to face-to-face visits to decrease patients' risk of contracting COVID-19. But for rural residents, telehealth was a double-edged sword. For some patients who had access to the internet, telehealth offered a way to seek treatment from their home. By receiving care at home, they did not have to drive the distance to the provider's office, eliminating travel time and cost. However, for patients who did not have access to the internet, telehealth offered additional challenges: They needed to either travel to a location where they had access to the internet, sometimes where there was no privacy, or they needed to postpone their visit or risk being seen in the provider's office.

Resilience

The COVID-19 pandemic devastated both short- and long-term commitments that nurses and other health care professionals had made for the protection of their patients and their own physical, behavioral, and spiritual health. From the winter of 2020 to the present day, nurses, in particular, have been faced with changes in their ideals of what their professional and personal lives should be and accept the realities of what their lives have become in this postpandemic world. In order to best understand these realities, one must examine the concepts of resilience and grit.

Resilience is an individual's ability to recover from stress (Munn et al., 2022). For instance, experiences such as failure to secure a promotion at work, stress associated with test taking, or fear of public speaking often can be overcome by practicing stress-reduction strategies. Grit interrupts an individual's long-term commitment toward goals (Munn et al., 2022). The loss of grit is a phenomenon that occurs over time. Unlike previous disasters, such as hurricanes, tornadoes, or threats of viral outbreaks (e.g., Avian flu), the COVID-19 virus caused a seismic shift in all aspects of our daily lives and resulted in a global crisis that continues to evolve. For nurses and health care providers, the consequences of this crisis have caused many to struggle, resulting in a loss of resilience and an erosion of personal grit.

According to Duckworth and Quinn (2009), culture has the power to shape our identity, what we expect of ourselves and what we are willing to change or not change because of who we are. Therefore, strategies that focus on self-care and self-actualization must be infused into nursing and health care curricula so that graduates enter the workforce informed and cognizant of their innate strengths to cope with both short- and long-term stressors.

Continuing education offerings, along with structured support networks, must be made available for nurses in all practice areas to lessen feelings of powerlessness and isolation. These networks, both virtual and face-to-face, will create vital linkages for nurses and health care staff and aid in both staff recruitment and retention. The question for nursing and health care leaders is if they are willing to provide the funding that will ensure these strategies remain in place for the long-term. "Gritty cultures help people develop their passion and require vision, relentless communication, experimentation, firmly embedded values and respect" (Meyer et al., 2019, p. 4).

Nurses have been aware of the need to establish a personal network for support for a long time. This comes from the isolation that is a result of living and working in rural settings. Networks allowing for the collaboration of nurses in rural areas were especially useful during the recent COVID-19 surges. These networks and resources should be replicated in geographic areas that provide care for marginalized rural communities to support health care providers in times of uncertainty and hardship.

Food Insecurities

Rural areas have been challenged with food insecurities for decades due to socioeconomic status and limited resources. There is a high number of rural children with food insecurities; many rural children receive both breakfast and lunch at school (Food Research & Action Center, 2018). One of the consequences of the pandemic was the closure of schools, leaving children without access to meals. In some areas across the United States, meals were available for families to pick up as needed. This did have a positive impact on feeding children, but it did not address the food insecurities that many have developed.

Workforce Shortages

Globally, there was a shortage of nurses and other health care providers before the pandemic; however, the pandemic has made the situation dire. Many health care workers left their positions due to having chronic illnesses that put them at high risk of illness if they contracted COVID-19, others left due to family demands, and others due to stress and fatigue. As the United States struggles with shortages of health care providers, with more profound shortages in rural areas (Table 17.1), strategies to ramp up recruitment and

TABLE 17.1 Per-Capita Rates of Health Professionals

Occupation	Health Professional per 10K, Rural	Health Professional per 10K, Urban
Dentist	4.7	7.6
Registered nurses	63.9	95.3
Licensed practical nurses/Licensed vocational nurses	21.8	18.4
Physician assistants	3.3	5.1
Physicians	12.7	33.6
Primary care physicians	5.2	8.0
Nurse practitioners	7.8	9.6
Total advanced practice registered nurses	10.0	12.7
Nurse anesthetists	1.3	1.8

Source Rural Health Information Hub (2024). Rural Healthcare Workforce:
https://www.ruralhealthinfo.org/topics/health-care-workforce

retention become more necessary. In rural areas, there is a limited number of providers to assist community members and other health care providers with the increased incidence in mental health challenges related to the pandemic. Due to limited physicians in rural areas, there has been an increase in the number of advanced practice registered nurses fulfilling the health care need. The shortage for registered nurses continues; there was a decrease from 11.98 nurses per 1,000 people in 2019 to 11.79 per 1,000 people in 2020 (Trading Economics, 2023).

Impact on Preventative Health and Cancer Screenings

Cancer screening involves a multistep process encompassing risk assessment, assessment, diagnosis, treatment, and surveillance (Croswell et al., 2021). In an effort to slow the spread of the COVID-19 virus, these procedures came to a sudden halt in the winter of 2020 when the U.S. government declared a cessation of all elective clinical procedures (Centers for Medicare and Medicaid, 2022). This declaration had both short- and long-term consequences for patients with known cancers (Patt et al., 2020). However, restrictions also included clinical procedures such as colonoscopies, prostate biopsies, computed tomography (CT), and cystoscopies that offer an opportunity to detect suspected or unexpected cancer (Englum et al., 2022). The suspension in access to care may have delayed identification of new cancers, leading to worse long-term outcomes (Turaga & Girota, 2020).

The cessation of diagnostic services has ended, and now health care providers must utilize this time as an opportunity to thoughtfully reassess cancer prevention programs and practices with the goal of lessening the health care disparities that exist in rural areas and their impact on marginalized high-risk cancer populations (Crosswell et al., 2021). An outcome of this process could be minimizing the overscreening of low-risk populations or those who may endure the physical and financial consequences from these interventions. Implementing these changes will require a change in practice that enhances health care inequities to practices that reduce historical disparities and positively impact cancer outcomes for all persons (Crosswell et. al, 2021).

Chronic Health Care

For families caring for a chronically ill child, COVID-19 made a difficult situation harder. The pandemic has highlighted the need for targeted psychosocial intervention for vulnerable families to address current mental health burdens and mitigate chronic psychological distress (McLoone et al., 2022). Researchers from Australia recruited parents of children receiving treatment for a chronic illness within the neurology, cancer, renal, and respiratory clinics at Sydney Children's Hospital. Some families reported feeling overwhelmed by the difficult decision of deciding whether to proceed with surgery, weighing the potential risks (exposure to COVID-19 within the hospital) and benefits (of surgery) for their child. Delays and cancellations of surgery due to hospital resources being depleted caused unimaginable anxiety among parents, as they watched their child's health deteriorate (McLoone et al., 2022). Figure 17.1 highlights the inter-relatedness of factors impacting families of children with chronic illness during the COVID-19 pandemic.

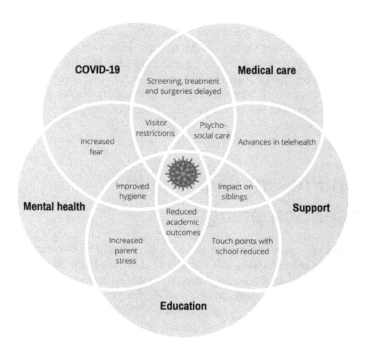

FIGURE 17.1 Inter-related factors impacting families of children with chronic illness due the COVID-19 pandemic.

McLoone et al. (2022) recommend the development of comprehensive models that offer a number of services, increasing in complexity as needed and addressing needs from diagnosis to disease progression and long-term care. Such programs are beginning to expand and grow in acceptance by families of these fragile children. One program model that is being expanded throughout Australia and Europe is called Contactless. This program is solely focused on the care needs of pediatric patients with rare and chronic conditions who typically need regular follow-up even in the absence of acute events. Contactless is a multifaceted, interdisciplinary telehealth model with an integrated framework for primary health care, with increased services based on need, up to the more complex levels of care (Mercuri et al., 2021).

Other vulnerable populations at risk from complications due to the COVID-19 virus are those at highest risk to experience severe complications, specifically rural elders over the age of 60 and those living with underlying health conditions such as cardiovascular and pulmonary disease or those with compromised immune systems (Bialek et al., 2020). There is a gap in the literature regarding prior potential epidemics, including the 2009 H1N1 influenza pandemic, as to whether public health information and education meets the needs of those at highest risk and if those individuals are more aware of their vulnerability, and if so, whether this translates to the initiation and maintenance of recommended protective actions.

In 2020, a team of researchers from the Greater Chicago area designed a study to examine the proactive practices of elders with chronic comorbidities to assess their likelihood to engage in preventative interventions (O'Conor et al., 2020). Data analysis from the study revealed that during the onset and initial spread of the COVID-19 virus, the majority of the 673 participants were able to identify the basic symptoms of COVID-19 and strategies they could take to minimize their risk of infection. There were no demographic differences in knowledge of COVID-19 symptoms or prevention strategies, yet fewer individuals reported taking steps to mitigate their risk of exposure, with only one third of individuals reporting social distancing practices (O'Conor et al., 2020). These findings emphasize the critical importance of concise and consistent public health messaging, across all communication platforms, to reach those at greatest risk of complications from infection (O'Conor et al., 2020). It is critically important for this vulnerable group to reconnect with health care providers who specialize in the care of older adults with chronic illnesses in order to return to a culture of proactive care management. As we move forward into the next phase of this pandemic, government and health care leaders must debrief in order to identify a national public health communication strategy that defines public health actions that allow and empower individuals to take preventive actions and feel that it is safe to return to health care providers in order to minimize their risks for emergent health needs.

The Shifting of Essential Personnel and Resources

The COVID-19 pandemic strained multiple U.S. health care systems. During the pandemic, the unprecedented spread of the COVID-19 virus and patients requiring care prompted many health care systems to reallocate resources and staff relocation to other areas. These changes impacted all specialty areas, including oncology whose patients were at increased risk due to being immunosuppressed (Anderson et al., 2021). At the onset of the COVID-19 pandemic, U.S. metropolitan communities demonstrated the highest incidence of the virus and the highest mortality. However, as the virus spread, higher incidence and mortality rates were evident in rural communities compared to urban areas (Andrews et al., 2021; Cuadros et al., 2021; Li et al., 2021, 2022). These rural–urban disparities in reaction to COVID-19 have been attributed to sparse health care resources (Peters, 2020), community opposition to the adoption of preventive measures (Islam et al., 2021), and vaccine hesitancy with lower vaccination rates (King et al., 2021) after vaccines became available.

Rural Health

Rural dwellers associate a state of health with the ability to work; to contribute to the family, community, or society; and to be able to perform common tasks without aid or assistance (Long & Weinert, 1989). Injustices in education, socioeconomic status, unemployment levels, lack of resources for financial stability for families, food insecurities, and other social determinants contribute to persistent health disparities between those living in America's rural and urban regions. In recent decades, differences between rural and urban Americans' life expectancy has grown, with rural residents dying on average 2 years earlier than their urban counterparts (Singh & Siapush, 2014; Figures 17.2 and 17.3). Rural communities face daunting challenges to access health care, health care services, and insurance compared to urban residents. The barriers for rural residents seeking rural health care have grown worse since the COVID-19 pandemic, and they present even greater challenges for these communities populated by rural dwellers who are older and sicker than they were prior to 2020.

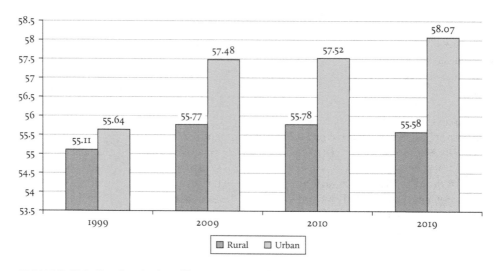

FIGURE 17.2 Rural and urban life expectancies for females.

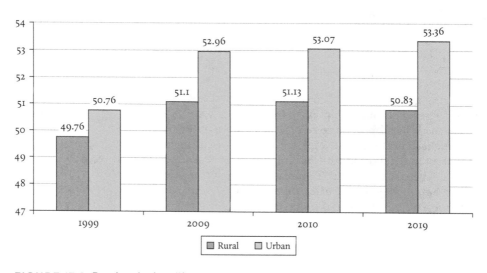

FIGURE 17.3 Rural and urban life expectancies for males.

According to the CDC (2023), "Residents in rural U.S. areas are more likely to die from heart disease, cancer, unintentional injury, chronic lower respiratory disease, and stroke than their urban counterparts. Unintentional injury deaths are approximately 50 percent (50%) higher in rural areas than in urban areas, partly due to greater risk of death from motor vehicle crashes and opioid overdoses" (para. 2). Figure 17.4 depicts efforts by the CDC to educate rural residents regarding their risks and strategies to mitigate those risks.

The CDC (2023) also stated that children in rural areas encounter greater challenges than urban children and that children in rural areas with mental, behavioral, and developmental disorders must overcome greater community and family challenges than children in urban areas with the same disorders. These challenges relate to geographic barriers, a shortage of pediatric health care providers in all areas, food insecurities, poverty, health literacy issues, and a lack of transportation and access to medical and psychiatric support. These

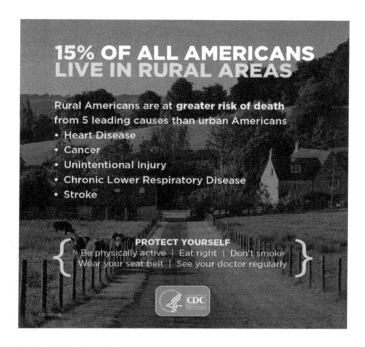

FIGURE 17.4 CDC poster.

challenges highlight the need for additional attention and resources aimed at improving health in rural America.

Rural areas could benefit from improved public health programs that support healthier behaviors and neighborhoods, and better access to health care services.

Availability, affordability, and acceptability have compounded the ability of rural people to access health care, health services, and health insurance for rural residents as compared to urban residents (Reilly, 2021). Moreover, rural hospital closures have reached crisis proportions since the COVID-19 pandemic. Figure 17.5 and Table 17.2 highlight 43 closures between 2005–2010 and 151 closures since 2010.

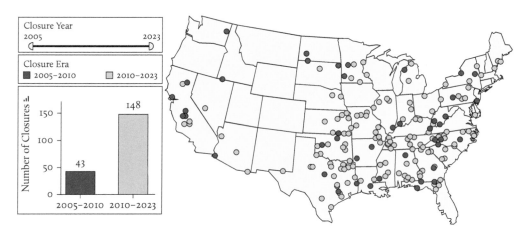

FIGURE 17.5 Rural hospital closures, 2005 to present.

Workforce Challenges

Workforce shortages posed significant challenges in rural areas for decades prior to the pandemic, and they became worse both during and after the pandemic. Twenty percent of the U.S. population is made up of rural communities, and they often are challenged by inadequate numbers of frontline health care providers and resources under nonemergency conditions. When CAHs reach capacity to provide care, rural hospitals and their communities may be faced with a reduction in access to critical care services and related resources because of time constraints and location, further exacerbating preexisting real and perceived health care disparities (Patel et al., 2021; Figure 17.6).

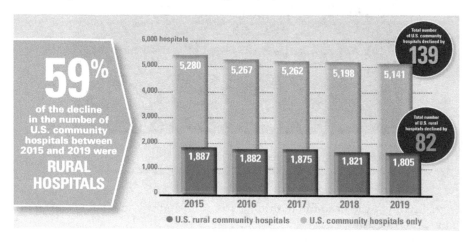

FIGURE 17.6. Decline in rural hospitals compared to community hospitals.

TABLE 17.2 Overview of Rural Hospital Closures

Year	Full Closures	Converted Closures	Total Closures
2010	1	2	3
2011	2	3	5
2012	5	4	9
2013	5	8	13
2014	8	8	16
2015	11	6	17
2016	5	5	10
2017	8	2	10
2018	9	5	14
2019	9	9	18
2020	10	9	19*
2021	0	2	2
Total	73	63	136

*The highest number of closure in a decade.

Source: University of North Carolina at Chapel Hill, The Cecil G. Sheps Center for Health Services (2023).

During the pandemic, rural hospitals supported one in 12 of the total rural jobs, adding $220 billion to the economics of rural communities (AHA, 2022). When a rural hospital closes, it has a large impact on the community. According to the University of North Carolina at Chapel Hill, The Cecil G. Sheps Center for Health Services Research (2023), from 2010 to 2021, 136 rural hospitals and health systems closed (Table 17.2).

Future Directions

As we approach nearly 5 years of living with the COVID-19 virus, it is important that health care systems and providers, leaders, and policymakers reflect on how the pandemic started, how it evolved, and what worked and what did not. We must learn from the devastation caused by the spread of COVID-19.

CASE STUDY 17.1

It is 2025, 5 years after the start of the COVID-19 pandemic. You are a student, and you are looking back at the impact of the pandemic. You are aware of the 1918 pandemic, and you have read some material on it and what changes were made to keep people safe. You have also read the material in this textbook and lived through the COVID-19 pandemic.

As you reflect on the past 5 years and look forward to the future, you realize that we need to learn from history, and you think about the changes to rural communities, the mental health of Americans, the financial state of the United States and the world, and what lessons we learned that we need to take forward to address the problems with our health care system and access to care.

Questions for Discussion Related to Case Study 17.1

1. What have Americans learned as a result of living through the COVID-19 pandemic?
2. Why hasn't there been a national debriefing focused on the COVID-19 pandemic?
3. Has the government stockpile of PPE been replenished? Will there be transparency in the allocation and distribution of these supplies?
4. What responsibilities do each of us bear in holding our policymakers and health care providers accountable for changes in public health practices?
5. How prepared will you be to emerge as a leader in nursing or health care to effectively address the next national or international crisis?

References

American Hospital Association. (2022). *Rural hospital closures threaten access: Solution to preserve care in local communities.* https://www.aha.org/system/files/media/file/2022/09/rural-hospital-closures-threaten-access-report.pdf

Anderson, M; Pitchforth, E; Asaria, M; Brayne, C; Casadei, B; Charlesworth, A; Coulter, A; Franklin, BD; Donaldson, C; Drummond, M; Dunnell, K;Foster, M; Hussey, R; Johnson, P; Johnston-Webber, C; Knapp, M; Lavery, G; Longley, M; Clark, JM; Majeed, A; McKee, M; Newton, JN; O'Neill, C; Raine, R; Richards, M; Sheikh, A; Smith, P; Street, A; Taylor, D; Watt, RG; Whyte, M; Woods, M; McGuire, A; Mossialos, E (2021). LSE-Lancet Commission on the future of the NHS: re-laying the foundations for an equitable and efficient health and care service after COVID-19. *The Lancet, 397*(10288), 1915–1978. 10.1016/S0140-6736(21)00232-4

Andrews, M. R., Tamura, K., Best, J. N., Ceasar, J. N., Batey, K. G., Kearse, T. A., Allen, L. V., Baumer, Y., Collins, B. S., Mitchell, V. M., & Powell-Wiley, T. M. (2021). Spatial clustering of county-level COVID-19 rates in the U.S. *International Journal of Environmental Research and Public Health, 18*, 1–22.

Bialek, S., Boundy, E., Bowen, V., Chow, N., Cohn, A., Dowling, N., Ellington, S., Gierke, R., Hall, A., MacNeil, J., Patel, P., Peacock, G., Pilishvili, T., Razzaghi, H., Reed, N., Ritchey, M., & Sauber-Schatz, E. (2020). Severe outcomes among patients with coronavirus disease 2019 (COVID-19)—United States, February 12–March 16, 2020. *Morbidity and Mortality Weekly Report, 69*(12), 343–346. https://doi.org/10.15585/mmwr.mm6912e2

Centers for Disease Control. (2023). *About rural health.* https://www.cdc.gov/ruralhealth/about.html

Centers for Medicare and Medicaid. (2020, April 20). *Non-emergent, elective medical services, and treatment recommendations.* https://www.cms.gov/files/document/cms-non-emergent-elective-medical-recommendations.pdf

Croswell, J. M., Corley, D. A., Lafata, J. E., Haas, J. S., Inadomi, J. M., Kamineni, A., Ritzwoller, D. P., Vachani, A., & Zheng, Y. (2021). Cancer screening in the U.S. through the COVID-19 pandemic, recovery, and beyond. *Preventive Medicine, 151*, 106595.https://doi.org/10.1016/j.ypmed.2021.106595

Cuadros, D. F., Branscum, A. J., Mukandavire, Z., Miller, F. D., & MacKinnon, N. (2021). Dynamics of the COVID-19 epidemic in urban and rural areas in the United States. *Annals of Epidemiology, 59*, 16–20. https://doi.org/10.1016/j.annepidem.2021.04.007

Duckworth, A. L., & Quinn, P. D. (2009). Development and validation of the Short Grit Scale (Grit-S). *Journal of Personality Assessment, 91*(2), 166–174. https://doi.org/10.1080/00223890802634290

Edwards, J. J., Wexner, S., & Nichols, A. (2021). *Debriefing for clinical learning.* Patient Safety Primer, Agency for Healthcare, Research and Quality. https://psnet.ahrq.gov/primer/debriefing-clinical-learning

Englum, B. R., Prasad, N. K., Lake, R. E., Mayorga-Carlin, M., Turner, D. J., Siddiqui, T., Sorkin, J. D., & Lal, B. K. (2022). Impact of the COVID-19 pandemic on diagnosis of new cancers: A national multicenter study of the Veterans Affairs Healthcare System. *Cancer, 128*(5), 1048–1056. https://doi.org/10.1002/cncr.34011

Food Research & Action Center. (2018). *Rural hunger in America: Gets the facts.* https://frac.org/wp-content/uploads/rural-hunger-in-america-get-the-facts.pdf

Islam, J. Y., Vidot, D. C., & Camacho-Rivera, M. (2021). Determinants of COVID-19 preventive behaviours among adults with chronic diseases in the USA: An analysis of the nationally representative COVID-19 impact survey. *British Medical Journal, 11*, e044600. https://doi.org/ 10.1136/bmjopen-2020-044600

King, W. C., Rubinstein, M., Reinhart, A., & Mejia, R. (2021). Time trends, factors associated with, and reasons for COVID-19 vaccine hesitancy: A massive online survey of US adults from January-May 2021. *PloS One, 16*(12), e0260731.https://doi.org/10.1371/journal.pone.0260731

Lakhani, H. V., Pillai, S.S., Zehra, M., Sharma, I., & Sodhi, K. (2020). Systematic review of clinical insights into novel Coronavirus (COVID-19) pandemic: Persisting challenges in

U.S. rural population. *International Journal of Environmental Research and Public Health*, *17*(12), 4279. https://doi.org/10.3390/ijerph17124279

Li, D., Gaynor, S. M., Quick, C., Chen, J. T., Stephenson, B. J. K., Coull, B. A., & Lin, X. (2021). Identifying U.S. county-level characteristics associated with high COVID-19 burden. *BMC Public Health*, *21*, 1007. https://doi.org/10.1186/s12889-021-11060-9

Li, Z., Lewis, B., Berney, K., Hallisey, E., Williams, A. M., Whiteman, A., Rivera-González, L. O., Clarke, K., Clayton, H., Tincher, T., Opsomer, J. D., Busch, M. P., Gundlapalli, A. V., & Jones, J. M. (2022). Social vulnerability and rurality associated with higher SARS-CoV-2 infection-induced seroprevalence: A nationwide blood donor study, United States, July 2020–June 2021. *Clinical Infectious Diseases*, *75*(1), e133–e143. https://doi.org/10.1093/cid/ciac105

Long, K. A., & Weinert, C. (1989). Developing the theory base. *Scholarly Inquiry for Nursing Practice: An International Journal*, *3*(2), 113–132.

McLoone, J., Wakefield, C. E., Marshall, G. M., Pierce, K., Jaffe, A., Bye, A., Kennedy, S. E., Drew, D., & Lingam, R. (2022). It's made a really hard situation even more difficult: The impact of COVID-19 on families of children with chronic illness. *PloS One*, *17*(9), e0273622. https://doi.org/10.1371/journal.pone.0273622

Mercuri, E., Zampino, G., Morsella, A., Pane, M., Onesimo, R., Angioletti, C., Valentini, P., Rendeli, C., Ruggiero, A., Nanni, L., Chiaretti, A., Vento, G., Korn, D., Meneschincheri, E., Sergi, P., Scambia, G., Ricciardi, W., Cambieri, A., & de Belvis, A. G. (2021). Contactless: A new personalised telehealth model in chronic pediatric diseases and disability during the COVID-19 era. *Italian Journal of Pediatrics*, *47*(1), 29. https://doi.org/10.1186/s13052-021-00975-z

Meyer, G., Shatto, B., Kuljeerung, O., Nuccio, L., Bergen, A., & Wilson, C. R. (2020). Exploring the relationship between resilience and grit among nursing students: A correlational research study. *Nurse Education Today*, *84*, 104246. https://doi.org/10.1016/j.nedt.2019.104246

Munn, A. C., George, T. P., Phillips, T. A., Kershner, S. H., & Hucks, J. M. (2022). Resilience and GRIT among undergraduate nursing students during the COVID 19 pandemic. *International Journal of Nursing Education Scholarship*, *19*(1). https://doi.org/10.1515/ijnes-2022-0012

O'Conor, R., Opsasnick, L., Benavente, J. Y., Russell, A. M., Wismer, G., Eifler, M., Marino, D., Curtis, L. M., Arvanitis, M., Lindquist, L., Persell, S. D., Bailey, S. C., & Wolf, M. S. (2020). Knowledge and behaviors of adults with underlying health conditions during the onset of the COVID-19 U.S. outbreak: The Chicago COVID-19 comorbidities survey. *Journal of Community Health*, *45*(6), 1149–1157. https://doi.org/10.1007/s10900-020-00906-9

Patel, L., Elliott, A., Storlie, E., Kethireddy, R., Goodman, K., & Dickey, W. (2021). Ethical and legal challenges during the COVID-19 pandemic: Are we thinking about rural hospitals? *The Journal of Rural Health*, *37*(1), 175–178. https://doi.org/10.1111/jrh.12447

Patt, D., Gordan, L., Diaz, M., Okon, T., Grady, L., Harmison, M., Markward, N., Sullivan, M., Peng, J., & Zhou, A. (2020). Impact of COVID-19 on cancer care: How the pandemic is delaying cancer diagnosis and treatment for American seniors. *Journal of Clinical Oncology Clinical Cancer Informatics*, *4*(4), 1059–1071. https://doi.org/10.1200/CCI.20.00134

Peters, D. J. (2020). Community susceptibility and resiliency to COVID-19 across the rural-urban continuum in the United States. *Journal Rural Health*, *36*, 446–456. https://doi.org/10.1111/jrh.12477

Reilly, M. (2021). Health disparities and access to healthcare in rural vs. urban areas. *Theory in Action*, *14*(2), 6–27. https://doi.org/10.3798/tia.1937-0237.2109

Rural Health Information Hub. (2024). *Rural Healthcare Workforce*. https://www.ruralhealthinfo.org/topics/health-care-workforce

Singh, G. K., & Siahpush, M. (2014). Widening rural-urban disparities in life expectancy, U.S., 1969–2009. *American Journal of Preventive Medicine, 46*(2), e19–29. https://doi.org/10.1016/j. amepre.2013.10.017

Trading Economics. (2023). *United States nurses.* https://tradingeconomics.com/united-states/ nurses

Turaga, K. K., & Girotra, S. (2020). Are we harming cancer patients by delaying their cancer surgery during the COVID-19 pandemic? *Annals of Surgery, 278*(5), e960–e965. https:// doi.org/10.1097/SLA.0000000000003967

University of North Carolina at Chapel Hill, The Cecil G. Sheps Center for Health Service Research (2023). *Rural Hospital Closures: 194 Rural Hospital Closures and Conversions since January 2005.* https://www.shepscenter.unc.edu/programs-projects/rural-health/ rural-hospital-closures/

World Population Review. (2023). *United States by density.* https://worldpopulationreview. com/state-rankings/state-densities

Image Credits

GLOSSARY

Affordable Care Act: Enacted in March 2010 (i.e., ACA, PPACA, or Obamacare), the law has three primary goals:

- Make affordable health insurance available to more people. The law provides consumers with subsidies ("premium tax credits") that lower costs for households with incomes between 100% and 400% of the federal poverty level (FPL).
- Expand the Medicaid program to cover all adults with income below 138% of the FPL. (Not all states have expanded their Medicaid programs.)
- Support innovative medical care delivery methods designed to lower the costs of health care in general.

American Rescue Plan: On January 20, 2021, President Joseph Biden passed the American Rescue Plan, an emergency legislative package aimed to fund vaccinations, provide immediate, direct relief to families bearing the brunt of the COVID-19 crisis, and support struggling communities.

Critical access hospitals: CAHs represent a separate provider type with their own Medicare conditions of participation (CoP) as well as a separate payment method. CAHs emerged to encourage states to strengthen rural health care options for both inpatient and outpatient services. They have more flexibility than other hospitals in staffing requirements.

Food insecurity: Defined as a condition of being unable to consistently have physical, social, and economic access to sufficient safe and nutritious food that meets dietary needs and food preferences for a healthy life.

Human trafficking: The U.S. Department of Homeland Security defines *human trafficking* as "trafficking involves the use of force, fraud, or coercion to obtain some type of labor or commercial sex act. Every year, millions of men, women, and children are trafficked worldwide—including right here in the United States. It can happen in any community and victims can be any age, race, gender, or nationality" (para. 1).

Personal protective equipment (PPE): PPE is equipment worn to minimize exposure to hazards that cause serious workplace injuries and illnesses. These injuries and illnesses may result from contact with chemical, radiological, physical, electrical, mechanical, or other workplace hazards.

Medically underserved: The U.S. Department of Health and Human Services defines *medically underserved areas/populations* as "areas or populations having too few primary care providers, high infant mortality, high poverty, or a high elderly population" (para. 2).

Public health emergency: The secretary of the U.S. Department of Health and Human Services (HHS) may, under section 319 of the Public Health Service (PHS) Act determine that (a) a disease or disorder presents a public health emergency or (b) that a public health emergency, including significant outbreaks of infectious disease or bioterrorist attacks, otherwise exists.

Telehealth: Telehealth—sometimes called telemedicine—lets your health care provider care for you without an in-person office visit. Telehealth is done primarily online with internet access on your computer, tablet, or smartphone.

REFLECTION

The final pages of this text are left blank for your reflections on the future of the world related to the COVID-19 pandemic, the lessons learned, and areas that need to be changed:

_____

_____

_____

_____

_____

_____

_____

_____

_____

_____

_____

_____

_____

_____

_____

_____

INDEX

loss of, 37
with worst three-year margins, 28–34
human trafficking, 65

I
illness and immunizations, 112–119
  case study, 115
  impact of vaccine hesitancy, 117–118
  nurse burnout, 113–115
  workplace health, 115–117
intensive care unit (ICU), 37
International Labour Organization (ILO), 60

J
Janke, A. T., 14
Jeitziner, M.-M., 147
Johnston, K. J., 42

K
Kim, J., 126
Kimhi, E., 126
Knighten, M. L., 114

L
Lathlean, J., 114
leadership, 125
  case study, 9
  complex relational, 10–11
  defined, 10
  executive, 11
  rural health, 2–6
  servant, 10
  styles, 9–11
  transactional, 10
  transformational, 9–10
  value of, during pandemic, 8–11
learner support, 106–110
  case study, 108
  nursing researchers, 107–108
  preventative approach, 109–110
  regulatory requirements, 106–108
Levett-Jones, T., 114
local health departments (LHDs), 51
Lowe, A. A., 50
Luna. P., 75

M
MacDonald, C., 148
Masha'al, D., 128

maternal health, 76–78
Maternal Telehealth Access Project, 77–78
Mauro, V., 54
McIlfatrick, S., 152
McLoone, J., 162
Medicaid payment rates, 53
medical-assisted treatment (MAT), 93
medical doctors (MDs), 43
medically underserved, 14–15
Medicare Rural Hospital Flexibility Program (Flex Program), 38
medication-assisted treatment (MAT), 55
Meleis, A. I., 131
mental health, 18
  health care workers and, 82–88
  of nurses, 85–86
  school-aged children, 98–99
mental health care
  access during crisis, 90–94
  case study, 94
  challenges and opportunities of referrals, 93–94
mental health treatment, 93
mentorship, 135–136
Mical, R., 117
Mine Safety and Health Administration (MSHA), 66
Modified Simulation Effectiveness Tool (SET-M), 128
Monnat, S. M., 119
Morin, K. H., 123
Mudallal, R. H., 113

N
National Association of School Nurses, 49
National Council Licensure Examination (NCLEX), 4, 122–123, 133–134
National Council of State Boards of Nursing (NCSBN), 3, 122, 133–134
National Emphasis Program (NEP), 68
National Health Service Corps (NHSC), 14–15, 136
National Institute for Occupational Safety and Health Epidemiologists, 66
National Institute on Aging (NIA), 147
National Labor Relations Board (NLRB), 135
National Rural Health Association, 119

National Rural Recruitment and
   Retention Network (3RNET), 134
National School Lunch Program (NSLP),
   100–101
Nease, D., 67
news articles, 51
nurse burnout, 113–115
Nurse Corps Loan Repayment programs,
   15
Nurse Licensure Compact, 3
nurse practitioners (NPs), 42
Nurses Corps Scholarship, 15
nursing education, 107–108
nursing practice, 122–129
   advocacy, 125
   case study, 124
   communication, 125
   core competencies for, 123
   critical thinking, 125
   flexibility, 125
   health policy, 125
   impact of COVID-19 pandemic on lives,
      128
   implications of COVID-19 pandemic for,
      123–124
   information and competencies for, 123
   international updates on use of simula-
      tion, 127–128
   leadership, 125
   new normal for, 125–126
   recommendations, 124
   simulation for preparing students,
      126–127
   teamwork, 125
nursing researchers, 107–108
nutrition, 100–102

O
Occupational Safety and Health
   Administration (OSHA), 60, 67–68
oncology, 75–76
opioid use disorder (OUD) treatment, 55

P
palliative and hospice care, 147–155
   data collection, 152
   decision-making, 149
   defined, 147
   findings, 150, 152
   impact of telehealth on, 154

outside of United States, 148
pediatric, 152–153
perceptions of rural dwellers regarding,
   150–151
quality between rural and urban community residents, 149–150
themes, 152
Panchuk, J., 148
Pathman, D. E., 135–136
Paycheck Protection Program (PPP), 39, 52
Pekince, H., 109–110
Perceived Stress Scale (PSS), 109
personal protective equipment (PPE), 2,
   52, 54
pharmacologic and nonpharmacologic
   treatments, 64
Phillips, K., 132
posttraumatic stress disorder (PTSD),
   82–83
primary and preventive health care, 64
primary care, 16
primary care provider (PCP), 42
Provider Relief Fund, 39
psychiatric mental health nurse
   practitioners (PMHNPs), 93
public health emergency, 37, 51
public health nurses (PHNs), 48–58
   case study, 50
   community health centers, 54–57
   defined, 48
   health department, 51
   home health settings, 51–54
   in United States, 48
   news articles, 51
   school nurse, 49–51

Q
quality health outcomes model (QHOM),
   149
Quinn, P. D., 159

R
registered nurses (RNs), 3
resilience, 159–160
Rural Development Broadband ReConnect
   Program, 22
Rural Emergency Acute Care Hospital
   (REACH) Act, 39
rural health/rural health care
   challenges and opportunities of, 14–25

Printed in the USA
CPSIA information can be obtained
at www.ICGtesting.com
LVHW060331270724
786416LV00024B/95

9 798823 303767